THIS IS NOT A DIET BOOK

Bee Wilson

THIS IS NOT A DIET BOOK

A User's Guide to Eating Well

4th ESTATE • *London*

4th Estate
An imprint of HarperCollins*Publishers*
1 London Bridge Street
London SE1 9GF
www.4thEstate.co.uk

First published in Great Britain by 4th Estate in 2016

1 3 5 7 9 8 6 4 2

A catalogue record for this book is
available from the British Library

ISBN 978-0-00-822576-6

Designed by BLOK www.blokdesign.co.uk

Printed and bound in Great Britain by
Clays Ltd, St Ives plc

MIX
Paper from
responsible sources
FSC **FSC® C007454**
www.fsc.org

FSC™ is a non-profit international organisation established to promote
the responsible management of the world's forests. Products carrying the
FSC label are independently certified to assure consumers that they come
from forests that are managed to meet the social, economic and
ecological needs of present and future generations,
and other controlled sources.

Find out more about HarperCollins and the environment at
www.harpercollins.co.uk/green

For David, who first taught me that balanced eating is less about health food and more about joy

CONTENTS

Introduction   2

Balance   12

How to Eat   36

What to Eat and Drink   54

Cooking   82

Children   106

Making Changes   132

Acknowledgements   146

RECIPES

A nourishing salad	20
Courgette spaghetti	32
Oatcakes to tide you over	44
Instant melon sorbet	69
Lentil soup for every season	73
My pho	91
Mushroom polenta	96
Tahini and black sesame porridge	97
Basil and lemon stew	99
Win–win waffles	114
Salad for a boy	122
Spiced chicken livers for a girl	126
Black bean chilli for a girl	128

THIS IS NOT A DIET BOOK

INTRODUCTION

There isn't time in the world to
examine all the food fads.
Logan Clendening,
The Balanced Diet, 1936

Most people hate diets, and who can blame us? Diets are generally the opposite of a good time. They leave you famished and force you to eat weird things that you don't enjoy. Diets dangle the promise of a new life – or a new body – only to make you feel like a failure when you can't stick to their insanely restrictive rules. Lose 6 pounds in six days on kale juice and walnuts and never feel hungry again! But you do feel hungry and, worse, you now feel guilty too.

Considering how unpleasant diets are – not to mention the fact that they generally leave us worse off than when we started – it's surprising how many of them we go on. Consumer research from 2013 suggested that more than half of all adults in Britain had tried to lose weight over the past year. The sad fact is that, much as we dislike dieting, we dislike our own bodies even more. Many of us are trapped in destructive eating habits. Given the broken food environment that now surrounds us, it's no wonder. It's hard to eat in a balanced way, when you have to walk a gauntlet of pink glazed doughnuts every time you go to the shops for milk. Yes, we are lucky to have access to abundant calories, something that many of our fellow citizens, in this country or elsewhere, still cannot rely on. But the distress of overeating – or believing that you are overeating – is also real.

As an overweight and self-loathing teenager, I was a sucker for diets. The Rotation diet, the F-plan diet, the 'don't eat anything except for celery and low-fat cream cheese until you nearly pass out' diet (this my own special invention). Each time I embarked on one, I felt I was slimming my way into a brave new dawn.

At gyms in January, you can see how desperate we can be for instant change. One morning last year, I saw a mother and her daughter – aged maybe 11 or 12 – weighing themselves before hitting the treadmills. An hour later, back in the changing room after a shower, I saw them weighing themselves for a second time, shaking their heads sorrowfully. The numbers on the scales had not gone down. Fail.

Our desire to change the way we eat can be so blinding it stops us from doing it. When you embark on a diet, you don't want slow and steady losses. You want to transform like a superhero. The fact that you have been here so many times before only makes it feel more urgent. Maybe *this* will be the one: the diet you can finally stick to. Such is the appeal of 'clean eating', the new form of dieting that pretends it isn't a diet. The idea is that if you fill your cupboard with enough packets of expensive chia seeds and gluten-free coconut flour, you can start afresh as a perfect person, someone who doesn't know the meaning of the words 'salted' or 'caramel'. You will *glow*. But then you accidentally eat a bagel. And since you are now officially dirty, you decide you might as well blow the whole thing and have two slices of chocolate fudge cake too. 'Clean eating' can't be the answer because food – unlike alcohol – isn't something you can go cold turkey on. Rather, we each have to find a way to make our peace with eating, in all its complexity.

'Eat food. Not too much. Mostly plants,' says food writer Michael Pollan. Wise words, but how on earth do you make yourself stick to them? It's not as if we don't already *know* that we should eat more plants and less food overall. But at some deep level, many of us don't want to do it. In 2013 more than half of British consumers surveyed (by Mintel) said that they didn't like diet food because the portions were too small.

Sometimes people say that our problem with food is that we are confused by all the competing information out there. Some experts tell us to avoid fat, while others insist we should avoid sugar. But when it comes to green leafy vegetables, the advice could hardly have been clearer. For decades, we have been told to eat more of them; and for decades, we have resisted. Only one in five people in Britain actually eats the recommended 'five-a-day' of vegetables and fruits according to a 2012 poll for the World Cancer

Research Fund. Rationally, we know we *should* eat more broccoli. But eating is far from rational.

Health campaigns fail for the same reason that diets do. They take no account of basic human psychology. We try to force ourselves to eat in a way that we don't like and are then disheartened when we find that we don't like it. A better way is to work to change our preferences themselves, until you become someone who enjoys the flavour of broccoli so much that you choose it of your own free will. Strange as it seems, this can be done. If you can make enough of these adjustments, you may never feel the urge to go on a diet again.

Asked on what occasions she drank champagne, the champagne heiress Lily Bollinger used to say that she drank it when she was sad and when she was happy; when she was alone and in company. 'Otherwise I never touch it – unless I'm thirsty.' I used to be the same with food. Any occasion, whether happy or sad, was a reason to gorge. And then there were times when I ate just because I was peckish. Which was pretty much always.

For many years, until my early twenties, my eating was chaotic and out of control. I would sit alone at the kitchen table eating whole pint-sized tubs of maple pecan ice cream. We talk in a sickly way of 'indulgent' foods, but when you are a compulsive eater, it does not feel like being pampered. Everywhere I went, food screamed at me. There were days and weeks when I gave myself up to consuming guilty treats. And then there were the not-eating phases, when I taunted myself with short-lived diets that started with raw carrots and hope and ended, a few days later, in pastries and despair.

I never thought I would end this futile cycle. But somehow, over a period of months, if not years, a happier way of eating crept up on me. Meal by meal, I reconditioned my responses to food. It was as if I were a child, learning how to eat all over again. Structure returned to my meals. Where once I'd hesitated to eat too heartily in public, in case someone thought me greedy, now I gave myself permission to eat until I was full. My tastes subtly altered. I found myself eating more vegetables, not to punish myself, but because they were – surprise! – delicious. I shrank from large to medium without really trying. This new life was the opposite of going on a diet.

My experiences are far from unique. Humans are more capable of improving their diets than we give ourselves credit for, as I discovered when doing the research for my last book, *First Bite*. We often speak in fatalistic and negative terms about our own eating, as if our taste for muffins and frappuccino were a life sentence. What we forget is that, as omnivores, we are extremely gifted at changing the way we eat to suit different environments. The consequences of bad diets are all around us, from type 2 diabetes to infant tooth decay. But the more research I did, the more encouraged I was to find that the scientific evidence suggests that our tastes and food habits are remarkably malleable. 'All of it is reversible,' as one senior doctor working with obese children put it to me. You could be cursed with all the genes that make a person susceptible to heart disease and obesity and still grow up healthy, by establishing balanced food habits.

This short book takes a rather different approach from *First Bite*, although it covers some of the same ground. I offer it to you as a sort of user's guide to eating. It is less about science or history and more about the practicalities of everyday life. Diet gurus often suggest that the answer to eating better is a return to the wisdom of grandmothers but my own hunch is that we need new skills to navigate this bewildering new world of food. We are the first generation to suffer more from plenty than want, and this changes everything.

How do we ditch the detox and find a way to want to eat what's good for us? How do we navigate the tricky questions of portion sizes and snacks? As a parent, how do you help your child to eat healthily, without becoming obsessive? How does anyone find a balanced way of eating that you can stick to for longer than two weeks? I kept thinking back to my own unhappy experiences with food and wanted to write something for other people who might feel similarly lost.

And yet I hesitate. What you put in your mouth is deeply personal. Bossy as I am (or so my children tell me), I'm not going to tell you what foods should pass your lips. I have no idea what you eat right now and whether it agrees with you or not. I can't see inside your fridge. I don't know your budget or your routines or whether you are overweight or underweight or whether you turn to food more in celebration or in sorrow. If you feel your eating – or not eating – is making you ill, a book – yes, even this one – is no substitute for professional help. One of the many problems with diet books is that they lay down the law, without pausing to consider the reader's personal circumstances. Maybe you are one of those lucky individuals – they do exist – for whom neither food nor weight has ever been an issue. If so, please tell me your secret.

I'm not going to prescribe any food laws, not least because when someone tells us what to eat, it's only natural to want to do the opposite. But in the course of eating for forty or so years, and feeding various people, including my own children, I feel I've learned some things that can make it all more of a joy and less of a struggle. These are the insights I wish I'd figured out sooner and hope you won't mind if I pass them on. I see them as tweaks more than rules. As you make your way through the book, feel free to ignore anything that doesn't apply to you.

This book can't give you a six-pack in seven days or the skin of a supermodel. But I can promise that if you make even a few of the adjustments in this book, your eating life will alter for the better in ways that you can sustain. The change that we are so desperate for *is* possible. Unlike a diet, these tweaks work with your appetites, rather than against them. I enjoy eating far more now than I ever did before, even though I am eating less. It's not about being thin – although for those who need it, long-term weight loss can definitely be achieved, no matter what people say. But the real end-goal is reaching the point where food is something that sustains you and gives you joy, rather than making you unhealthy or unhappy.

You know you have changed when the new habits start to be automatic and the old clamour of guilt and indulgence is switched off. One day, you eat a platter of fresh and vibrant greens with soy sauce and garlic, not because you think you should or because it's January but because it happens to be what you feel like eating at that precise moment. In this new life, a life beyond diets, there is no fail.

BALANCE

That kind of health which can be preserved only by a careful and constant regulation of diet is but a tedious disease.

Attributed to Montesquieu

1

The only diet worth going on is the one you never have to come off.

2

The major obstacle to changing your diet is in some ways the most obvious one: no one – adult or child – likes eating foods that they do not like. Our challenge is therefore to enjoy new ways of eating. You won't find the miracle cure in any product that you can buy, whether it's probiotics or seaweed. The answer is in your own brain. If you feel trapped in unhealthy ways of eating, you need to reboot some of your tastes until you are consoled and excited by different foods.

3

Eating in a balanced way doesn't mean every meal has to be nutritionally 'perfect' (not that there is such a thing, in any case). A balanced diet could mean spinach and chickpea soup for lunch but spaghetti carbonara for dinner. The journalist Mark Bittman lost a substantial amount of weight and improved his health by eating as a vegan before 6 p.m. and then anything he fancied for the rest of the day (as he explains in his book *VB6*). Balance means taking pleasure in many different foods. An obsession with making every plate immaculately balanced can itself become unhinged. The great American food writer M.F.K. Fisher once lamented the trend for combining 'a lot of dull and sometimes actively hostile foods' in a single meal, purely for the sake of covering your nutritional bases. Fisher wisely wrote: 'Balance the day, not each meal in the day.'

4

One person's health food is another's poison. It would be genuinely impossible to construct a balanced diet to suit everyone. Don't take your cues about what to put in your body from someone else's needs. There's so much noise and nonsense about diet that needs to be filtered out. A celebrity may – in all honesty – attribute her good looks and health to the fact that she avoids 'nightshades' such as tomatoes. An endurance runner may insist that the secret of his success is 2 litres of chocolate milk a day. But avoiding tomatoes and drinking large amounts of chocolate milk may not work quite such wonders for you.

5

Diets like to pretend that certain foods are absolutely good or absolutely bad. The truth is messier. If you are asking, 'How much should I eat?' of any given food, the answer is somewhere between 'at every meal' and 'never'. In Overeaters Anonymous, recovering overeaters divide foods up into 'red', 'green' and 'amber'. 'Red' foods are ones that you decide never to eat (a junk food meal of hamburger, fries and milkshake, let's say). 'Green' foods are ones you will eat without limits (vegetables). All the other foods – from macadamia nuts to fajitas – occupy the in-between state of 'amber', to be eaten 'in moderation'. All of us – overeaters or not – have to find a way to live and eat in a state of amber.

6

Your first job when eating is to nourish yourself. Food can be many things: it can be entertainment, culture and even art. But unless it is sustenance – something that keeps you alive and gives you energy and strength – it is not food. Example: a 10-calorie pot of low-calorie 'fruit' jelly – zero fat, zero protein, almost zero carbohydrate – is not really food. Among other lost eating skills – see also How to Eat, below – we seem to have lost the basic and old-fashioned concept of 'nourishing' ourselves. You can be overweight and still not getting enough good food to eat – in fact, plenty of people are. Around the world, obese populations suffer disproportionately from micronutrient deficiencies, notably vitamins A and D, plus zinc and iron. Junk foods may be high in calories but they are low in nourishment. Learning how to eat better is not about reducing consumption across the board. While we undoubtedly need to eat less of many foods – sugar springs to mind – we need more of others.

7

Calories are not the same as morals. No food can be either 'naughty' or 'virtuous'. Cheesecake is not sin. It's all just food. I'm not saying that everything for sale is worth putting in your mouth. Whole sections of the supermarket are now devoted to products that don't deserve the name of food at all. We'd all do well to avoid these non-foods, as far as possible. But this isn't a question of individual morals. If anyone should feel sinful, it's the manufacturers who cynically push these fake, sugar-laden products at us without any regard for what they will do for our health. The end-goal here isn't to 'be virtuous' but to adjust your tastes and habits – or enough of them – so that the overall pattern of what you eat consists of real foods, especially plant foods, eaten in regular instalments and with pleasure. If you manage to do this, the calories will take care of themselves.

8

Sugar is not love. But it can feel like it.

Don't feel bad because you crave a little sweetness occasionally (OK, every day). This isn't a moral defect; it's human nature. A love of sweet tastes is hard-wired in babies the world over, from China to Denmark. What makes sweetness feel even more wonderful is that the first food any of us knows is milk, which is both sweet and given to us along with the cradling warmth of a parent. From our earliest tastes, we receive sweetness and love together, so we could be forgiven if later in life we have trouble distinguishing the two. During my first term at university, I sometimes sat alone in my student room, sipping Diet Coke and eating compulsive handfuls of jelly beans, wishing I could leave the room and meet someone but feeling unable to do anything about it.

A big part of learning to eat better is unravelling the connection between sweets and love. When you use sugar as an emotional prop, there is no reason to stop. No ice cream, no matter how caramel-intense, will satisfy your hunger if what you really wanted was friendship or to be touched.

9

Eating well is a skill. We learn it. Or not. It's something we can work on at any age. The three big things we would all benefit from learning to do are: following structured mealtimes; responding to our own internal cues for hunger and fullness rather than relying on external cues such as portion size; and making ourselves open to trying a variety of foods, especially vegetables. All three of these skills can and have been taught to children; and we adults can learn them too, if we give ourselves the chance.

10

If you sometimes feel a little overwhelmed by the process of choosing what to eat for the best, and how to stick at it, join the club. No generation has ever had to navigate a world of such bewildering plenty as the one we now inhabit. We live in an environment pretty much engineered to make us a) overeat and b) have complicated emotions about food. Sometimes glib people tell us that eating well is incredibly simple and that *all* we have to do to be healthier is 'eat less and move more'. Thanks, Einstein! Actually, neither part of this irritating saying is true. Exercise by itself doesn't seem to generate weight loss (although it's still pretty much essential for lots of other reasons: see Making Changes below). Simply *eating less* by itself is also not the answer. A smaller quantity of junk food is still junk and calories are never the whole story. Calories alone do not tell you how easily the microbes in your gut will cope with this or that particular food, or what it will do to your blood sugar or whether the flavour will trigger you to eat three helpings of it. More to the point, if it were so very simple to 'eat less and move more', we'd all be doing it.

11

Judge food by what it has in it – not by what it doesn't. So many packaged foods boast about what they have taken out: 'free from' this, 'no added' that. Zero per cent fat, reduced sugar, reduced salt. These terms are usually just marketing devices trying to persuade us to spend good money on bad food. Perhaps more damaging, they are part of a wider mindset that views healthy eating in fundamentally negative terms, as something that doesn't have anything supposedly 'bad' in it.

A NOURISHING SALAD

Back when I was unhappy about food, I thought I should eat salads precisely because they had almost nothing in them. I thought of nutrition as a form of absence. Fat-*free*, sugar-*free*. At the height of the low-fat craziness of the 1990s, my best friend C and I (she was a recovering anorexic) used to sit side by side chomping through salads containing little but dull iceberg lettuce, over-refrigerated tomatoes and possibly half of a pallid chicken breast. No dressing, no flavour, no joy.

Now that my relationship with eating has changed, I see that what makes salads great is that you can fit so much nourishment and variety into a single easy plateful (or Tupperware box). A salad is a vehicle for good things like toasted nuts, bright herbs, juicy roasted vegetables and cheese. Depending on the time of year, it might be leftover charred peppers with aubergine purée and feta; or roasted pumpkin with sage, pearl barley, hazelnuts and watercress. Some torn-up chicken from yesterday's roast dinner might make a welcome second appearance with black grapes, cucumber, mint and rice, rather tartly dressed. Whatever the time of year, I like carrot salads, both raw and cooked: great for when you feel broke but in need of zingy sustenance (even organic carrots are cheap). Canadian food writer Naomi Duguid makes an incredible Burmese carrot salad with peanuts, lime juice, fish sauce and fried shallots. Steamed sliced carrots dressed with oil, garlic, lemon and chopped coriander is another good way.

But my new favourite involves toasted cumin seeds and currants and is loosely based on something I ate at a marvellous café in Portland, Oregon, called Maurice Luncheonette (the version there contained prunes). I've added torn chunks of garlicky toast, as a nod to the legendary chicken and bread salad in *The Zuni Café Cookbook*, and to make it filling enough for lunch.

If the word salad has bad connotations for you, do as food writer Sally Butcher does and call it a 'salmagundi' instead (an old name for a mixture of many ingredients). In fact, call it whatever you like.

Carrot and bread salad:
a nourishing but cheap lunch

Serves 3

1 tablespoon currants

2 teaspoons apple cider vinegar (I like the one made
    by Raw Health)

2 tablespoons pumpkin seeds

2 teaspoons cumin seeds

2 tablespoons extra virgin olive oil

4 spring onions, chopped

750g carrots

3 generous slices sourdough bread

1 clove garlic

sea salt (preferably Maldon)*

20g flat-leaf parsley, chopped

* I use Maldon sea salt, a teaspoon of which has half as
much sodium as a teaspoon of free flowing fine salt, because
it is less dense; in general, if you are using regular salt, you
will only need half the amount.

Put the currants in a small bowl and pour over the vinegar. Heat up a wide large pan or skillet and toast the pumpkin seeds until some of them pop. Tip into a bowl. Add the cumin seeds to the pan for a couple of seconds until fragrant. Set them aside with the pumpkin seeds. Heat 1 tablespoon of the oil and soften the spring onions for a minute or two. Peel the carrots and trim off the ends. Using a food processor, cut half the carrots into wafer-thin slices and grate the other half. If you don't have a food processor, grate half the carrots on a box grater and slice the others as thinly as you can, with a peeler or a knife. Meanwhile, toast the bread in the toaster, rub the cut clove of garlic all over it and drizzle the second tablespoon of oil over the slices. Sprinkle the toast with salt and cut or tear into 2cm chunks. Now mix all the ingredients together and season again with salt, to taste. Add more vinegar or a squeeze of lemon if you think it needs it. I like this with fish; but it's a good lunch all by itself.

12

Our lives would be more balanced if we spent less time worrying about our weight and more time planning what to cook for dinner. How much better we would eat if we took all those hours of unhappy weight-obsessing and diverted them to dreaming up different uses for herbs (you haven't lived until you've tried a deep-fried sage leaf).

13

A word about guilty pleasures: there is no such thing (and don't get me started on 'guilt-free' snacks). If it's making you feel guilty, it isn't a pleasure. And pleasure in eating is nothing to feel ashamed of, whatever your size. One of the saddest things about our eating today is the way we have been conditioned to sabotage our own joys. Shame never made a person eat better. When you think that eating cake is a cause for shame, you are likely to eat it in secret and in much larger quantities (I write from experience). Give yourself permission to eat such things in limited quantities but without guilt and you may discover, to your surprise, that one occasional slice, eaten with gusto and joy, is enough.

14

If you want to change your diet long-term – and lose weight, if you need to – change your tastes. I recently met someone who had lost nearly 100 pounds over the course of a year. 'How has it been?' I asked her, half expecting her to say, as so many dieters do, that it had been torture. 'Oh, it's been marvellous,' she said. 'I'm having a wonderful time changing my palate.' This may be an extreme reaction (and you might not share it). But long-term studies confirm that people who successfully lose a lot of weight without regaining it – these people are known as 'maintainers' – tend to say their appetites have permanently changed. These people seem to actually enjoy their food more than the dieters who relapse. The relapsers feel that when 'on a diet' they should forbid themselves anything they enjoy. By contrast, the maintainers never completely restrict their old comfort foods, but as time went by, they changed the way they cook, making smaller portions and eating more vegetables and grains. But the real change is to themselves, because this is how they now want to eat.

15

We all start from a different place with food. You didn't choose the genetic cards you were handed when it comes to the way you eat. Maybe you are a supertaster, someone for whom bitter flavours taste incredibly strong. Or maybe you were born with genes that predisposed you to anorexia or pickiness. There is a strong genetic component to many eating disorders; and also to obesity. Scientists working with twins have found that, eating a very similar diet, one twin may gain weight while the other doesn't, purely due to differences in their gut microbes. Life is unfair. But wherever we start, it's possible to develop new tastes and new habits.

16

You are not doomed to eat badly. The overall pattern of how we eat is governed more by environment than biology. This helps explain why we are in such a mess with our diets now because no one has ever had to learn how to eat in such a toxic food world as the one we now inhabit. Every day, we are bombarded with confusing messages that tell us it is normal to eat in dysfunctional ways. It sometimes feels as if our appetites were not our own. But the good news is that, if our tastes are largely formed by environment, then it's also possible to change them, under the right circumstances. There is nothing innate in your physiology that says you will always prefer hamburgers to ratatouille.

17

If food habits are learned, they can also be relearned. Most of us have a firm belief that our likes and dislikes are part of our personality, something we are powerless to change. Social media only makes it worse, because we project our food tastes to the world. We announce: I am a chocoholic, a carnivore or a cheese-addict, and it becomes a badge of honour, a deep part of who we are. Entire relationships have been founded on a mutual loathing for liquorice. But imagine you were adopted at birth by liquorice-loving parents who lived in a remote village in a far-flung country. Your tastes would be quite different from the ones you ended up with. Even now, you can adjust your preferences. The only downside is that you may have to change your Facebook status.

18

Nothing tastes good when it's eaten in a spirit of coercion. The secret is – as far as possible – to make healthy food and pleasurable food one and the same.

Our culture tends to put health food and enjoyable food in two separate boxes. Health food is 'eat up your greens' and puritanism. When I used to go on diets, I felt ravenous before I'd even eaten the first breakfast because I was 'on a diet'. The last thing I wanted to eat was whatever the particular diet was advising. It didn't have much to do with the food itself. It was a state of mind.

I overheard a woman in a café chatting to a friend over weekend lattes and eggs Benedict about her attempts to adopt a healthier lifestyle. She announced that, on Monday, she was going to buy kale and make green juice. 'The trouble is, I buy the kale, it sits in the fridge, I throw it away. I buy it again, throw it away again.' I related to what she was saying. When you think that kale is something you need to swallow as a form of self-improvement, it tastes vile.

But what if you properly liked kale? Then, it would be easy to eat. After buying the kale, the next step is to try the kale. Offer it kindly. Coax yourself with small morsels. Pair it with other foods that you like (the dark mineral taste goes well with chorizo, or as a purée stirred through pasta). Or crisp it in the oven with oil and salt, as if it were chips. One day, you may find yourself eating a plate of kale with bright oil and garlic and two poached eggs, not because you feel you should, or that it will make you a better person, but because you positively crave it, especially black kale (cavolo nero) which is not as scratchy as curly kale. Then again, you may never warm up to kale and its stalky charms. No matter. There are always other foods.

19

Try to start thinking of feeding yourself as a good parent feeds a child: with love, with variety, but also with limits.

As adults, so many of us feed ourselves in ways that are alternately neglectful and overly strict: first, we let ourselves eat a whole family-size bag of crisps with a bucket-sized glass of wine but then we deny ourselves lunch. Next time you sit down to eat, imagine you are an ideal parent feeding a beloved child. Wouldn't it be nice if you could offer yourself food in a warm, structured, no-fuss kind of way? You wouldn't punish yourself with crash diets but nor would you allow yourself too much junk. Your priority when choosing food would be to see yourself well nourished and you'd choose meals to keep your mood on an even keel. You'd want yourself to enjoy eating. The fridge would be stocked with good food and you would trust yourself to choose wisely from its contents.

20

Stop being cruel to yourself about eating. You are not 'naughty' because you broke your stupid diet and ate some pasta. You are a human body needing to be fed. We should be far less judgemental about ourselves and our eating habits and far more judgemental about the diets that make us feel like losers for preferring a bowlful of comforting tagliatelle to one of spiralized courgette.

'Courgetti' – an approximation of spaghetti made from raw ribbons of courgette – is an example of how crazy and extreme our ideas of diet have become. If you want to spiralize vegetables, be my guest. The telephone-wire texture of spiralized vegetables has its appeal, and it's fun to watch the strands tumble from the spiralizer. But pasta it is not. Replacing your usual plate of refined white pasta with a pile of vegetable mush will not make you 'glow'. It will make you hungry, and then you start to feel like a failure when you crave a huge bowl of cereal an hour after dinner. Instead of giving you the absurd choice of courgettes *or* pasta, a kinder diet might lead you towards courgettes *and* pasta, but with more vegetables and fewer noodles.

Diet books are always nagging you to eat wholewheat pasta, which is OK once in a while (there's a Nigella recipe for spelt pasta with anchovies that I love) but if you have it too often it can feel like chewing on cardboard. Do as the Italians do and enjoy refined white durum-wheat pasta but in smaller quantities. We are doing pasta a disservice when we dismiss it as a beige 'carb' with no redeeming features. An 85g serving of De Cecco egg pappardelle contains 11g of protein. Even non-egg dried pasta contains at least 8g of protein per portion, depending on portion size and brand.

When I cook pasta and vegetables now, I measure the pasta sparingly and add quantities of greens that I would once have thought excessive. I've come to prefer it that way, assuming the vegetables are well-seasoned and treated with care. Sometimes, at home, we eat two whole heads of cauliflower between five, broken up and sautéed in oil with shallots until brown and crispy, then tossed with farfalle, olives and toasted breadcrumbs. Other times, I make penne with overcooked broccoli, a deeply comforting recipe borrowed from Jacob Kenedy's *The Geometry of Pasta*, in which the broccoli cooks with the pasta in its water before being tossed with garlic-scented reduced cream. Or we eat versions of this courgette pasta, which is so much better than courgetti.

Courgette spaghetti (not courgetti)

The grated courgettes cook down to a deliciously melting consistency. I add peas at the end, for a different texture, and sweetness.

Serves 4–5

500g courgettes

3 tablespoons extra virgin olive oil

½ teaspoon Maldon sea salt

a pinch of chilli flakes

2 cloves garlic

200g frozen petits pois

zest of 1 lemon and juice to taste

nutmeg

400g spaghetti

Parmesan or pecorino

Bring a large pan of water to the boil. Meanwhile, grate the courgettes. Warm the oil in a large wide frying pan or skillet. Add the courgettes, salt and chilli flakes. Cook gently, turning with a wooden spoon, until they start to soften. Add the garlic cloves, finely sliced, and stir for a few minutes more until very soft and tender. Stir in the peas for a minute or two until just defrosted. Add the zest and juice of the lemon – start with the juice of half the lemon – and a grating of nutmeg (if you like). Taste to see if it needs more salt. Cook the spaghetti – with plenty of salt in the water – according to the instructions on the packet. Drain the spaghetti, reserving a cup of cooking water. Mix the pasta and courgettes, adding as much of the cooking water as you need to loosen the sauce. Serve with Parmesan if you like (I do, but without the Parmesan, this is something you could serve to a vegan friend, perhaps adding toasted pine nuts instead).

21

Break the old associations. If you are picky about healthy foods, try to identify exactly what it is about the food that you find off-putting. Maybe porridge reminds you of the lumpy semolina you were given as a child; or maybe you can't abide cauliflower because it takes you back to eating watery cauliflower cheese. Try to introduce yourself to new dishes with fresh connotations. I recently met a man who had lost (and kept off) a huge amount of weight, after more than a decade of being obese. He said he had always hated vegetables because of school dinners. When he tasted carrots, no matter how nicely cooked they were, he was reminded of those soggy orange chunks in the school canteen. What finally made him change his diet was the realization that he was allowed to eat vegetables that didn't exist in the Britain of his youth. Now, he eats red peppers and sugarsnap peas; butternut squash and rocket and mizuna, which no dinner lady ever forced him to swallow.

HOW TO EAT

It is only the dose which makes
a thing poison.
*Paracelsus (Philip von
Hohenheim), Third Defence from
The Seven Defences of Paracelsus*

1

Before you change what you eat, change *how* you eat. It is virtually impossible to have a healthy relationship with food if you don't eat structured meals, with gaps in between. Many of us – whatever our size – relate to food in chaotic ways, hurtling through the day without ever quite eating what you could call an actual meal. For some (this was my life), the chaos takes the form of compulsive overeating. For others, the chaos is not eating enough, whether because of anorexia, dieting, or extreme picky eating. Some 'clean eaters' are so obsessed with the purity of what they put in their mouths that they dare not accept invitations to eat with friends. This is no way to live. Other people skip meals through sheer busyness, because there are so many supposedly more 'important things' to get through in the lunch hour that lunch itself is forgotten.

Whatever the reason for the chaos, the first step in eating better is to work to weave structured meals into your day, if you haven't already done so. No starving, no bingeing (although slip-ups will happen and that's OK; in earlier, more generous times, such slip-ups were called 'feasts'). There are no prizes for being the person who didn't eat dinner.

2

Reclaim breakfast, lunch and dinner. This is the first and most important change you can make. So many of our anxieties around diet take the form of a search for the perfect food, the one that will cure all our ills. Should you buy a super-expensive high-speed blender and drink green juice every morning? Should you get a special high-omega seed mix and scatter it like unction on everything you consume? Don't let me stop you, if green juice and seeds are your thing. But no miracle product can possibly be as effective a diet tool as the simple act of giving yourself permission to eat regular, modestly sized meals, preferably sitting at a table, with predictable gaps of no-eating in between.

3

As you move from chaos to structure, don't feel you need to change the substance of what you eat too radically. Have anything you like for these meals – you could even choose cake with berries and whipped cream for breakfast, if that's what thrills you. You will still be feeding yourself better than you were before, if your eating patterns were chaotic. Bit by bit, you will probably find that your tastes change and the nutritional quality of what you eat improves all of its own accord just through sticking to regular meals, because not many people choose doughnuts for dinner or crisps for breakfast (though as someone who would once start the day with Pickled Onion flavour Monster Munch, I know that it can be done).

4

Treat your meals as if they are worth the trouble of eating; and treat yourself as if you deserve to eat them.

5

Build new rituals into your eating. Aim to eat your meals at roughly the same time each day until you condition yourself to expect food at certain times and not at others. Pay more attention to the food on your plate; try to be fed by the colours and textures as much as by the flavours. Dignify your eating with some of the paraphernalia of dining, even when you are forced to eat away from a table. In the children's book, *Bread and Jam for Frances*, the main character carries a doily and a small vase of violets in her school lunchbox and lays it out before she eats. I'm not suggesting you go this far. But if you are stuck eating breakfast on a train, say, buy yourself the nicest coffee flask you can afford and carry a jam jar layered with yoghurt, berries and toasted nuts and a proper spoon to eat it with; or some comforting slices of warm wholegrain toast in a brown paper bag, with a pat of butter and a tiny knife for spreading, if you have enough elbow room to do this on your commute.

6

Map out the full contents of a meal before you take the first mouthful. It helps if you can think, This is what there is and this is all there is, rather than treating your food cupboards and fridge as a continuous smorgasbord that you can keep dipping into. But when deciding your meals, be generous, not stingy. Give yourself small rewards every day, whether it's a little piece of nougat after lunch, a particularly delicious peach or a glass of Prosecco.

7

If you have to eat lunch at work, consider buying a bento box. The original Japanese bento was pioneered using aluminium boxes in the early twentieth century and offers a structure ideally designed for eating a healthy lunch. Rectangular compartments are filled with varied flavours, artistically arranged: rice, vegetables, protein (tofu or fish, some chicken skewers or a Japanese omelette) and beautiful fruit. But I find you can adapt the bento idea and put pretty much anything in that box, ranging from yesterday's leftover stir-fry to cold curry and rice (nicer than it sounds if you add a wedge of lemon and coriander leaves) to Middle Eastern meze and any kind of hearty salad of roasted vegetables and grains.

A bento box – or the equivalent size of any sealed plastic box – gives an easy handle on portion sizes, without any need to count calories or obsess about nutrients. If you only consume what is in your bento it should be impossible to overeat. Conventionally in Japan, the sizes are 300ml for little kids, 600ml for adults with 'modest' appetites and 900–1,000ml for hearty eaters, but I found that the Japanese idea of a 'modest' portion was my idea of microscopic. If you have a bento with many compartments it will also encourage you to eat a greater variety of foods – especially vegetables – to fill them up. When you get the structure of eating right, the rest falls into place.

8

If it's not a mealtime and you are wondering which of two 'healthy' snacks you should buy, the answer is probably neither.

If it is a mealtime, and you are vacillating between two main courses, go for the one you really love, the one you think will satisfy you the most. And when you are full, stop.

9

Plan your snacks. If you feel you need more than three meals a day – and many of us clearly do – then make them a regular part of the day, just like your other meals, rather than being endlessly derailed by them. Food writer Meera Sodha notes that 'no Indian mother ever taught her child not to snack between meals' because snacks, from kachori stuffed with peas to spicy savoury chaat of various kinds, are a fully integrated part of the food culture in India. Recovering anorexia sufferers work to eat three meals and three snacks a day. It sounds a lot but most of us eat far more than that, with mouthfuls here and there that we hardly notice or enjoy.

The French have a delightful ritual called *le goûter* – a moment after school when children pause for something like a piece of bread with dark chocolate and a glass of milk. This is worth copying. If you know you get ragingly hungry at 4 p.m. every day, you may as well prepare for it. Most snack foods get to you because you buy them on impulse – whether the supposedly 'healthy' ones masquerading as something high in protein or fruit or the obviously 'unhealthy' ones loaded with sugar, refined oils and salt. Much better to carry your own provisions and decide in advance what you will eat when hunger strikes. There are times when only a cake or cookie will do. These are afternoons to enjoy. Don't spoil the pleasure of the cake with guilt. But most days you might want to choose something that delivers less of a sugar rush.

SOME GOOD SNACKS

A crisp apple or juicy nectarine
A handful of almonds and a couple of squares of dark
    chocolate
A hard-boiled egg with Maldon sea salt, pepper and
    celery sticks
Crunchy carrots and guacamole
Two corn cakes slathered with nut butter
Home-made samosas
Cheese and grapes
Good toast with ricotta, honey and sliced figs
Oatcakes

Oatcakes to tide you over

These were inspired by a recipe by food writer
Felicity Cloake in her column in the *Guardian*. Her
version uses three different varieties of oats. The
texture is excellent, but I'm not usually quite
organized enough for the shopping, so I've
compromised by whizzing half the oats in the food
processor and leaving half whole. My recipe uses
olive oil instead of Cloake's butter. These oatcakes are
so much better than any you can buy and are also
excellent with cheese. You could make them gluten-
free with gluten-free oats (check the packet) and they
are also good for people who can't eat yeasted bread.
It's well worth doubling the recipe. They keep for a
week in a tin.

Makes 12–15
300g jumbo oats, preferably organic
¼ teaspoon Maldon sea salt
1 teaspoon brown sugar
75g extra virgin olive oil
75ml boiling water

Line a couple of trays with baking parchment. Preheat the oven to 200°C. Put the oats on one of the trays and bake for 10–15 minutes or until toasty. Allow to cool slightly. Measure out half the oats (150g) and whizz to a fine powder in the food processor. Add the salt, sugar, oil and boiling water from a kettle and whizz again. Finally add the second half of the oats and pulse to a dough (don't overmix). Roll it out about ½ centimetre thick and cut into rounds. How many you get will depend on the size of your cutter and how thick you rolled the dough, but don't worry, I've made these in varying sizes and they always come out well. Place on the trays and bake for 20 minutes. Carefully turn with a fish slice and return to the oven for another 5–10 minutes. Leave to cool on their trays for a couple of minutes before carefully transferring to a wire rack to cool completely.

NB – If you don't have a food processor, you can substitute half of the oats with ready-ground oatmeal and mix the dough by hand in a mixing bowl.

10

Learn to recognize – and act on – the feeling of being satisfied by food and try, hard as it is, to be satisfied with less. Just as it is possible to learn to enjoy new tastes, you can train yourself to enjoy new levels of fullness until that old sensation of tightness around the belt is actively unpleasant. This process of learning new levels of fullness is especially tricky if you were brought up – as I was – to leave a clean plate. David Kessler, an American doctor, recommends experimenting with eating half your usual portion of lunch and then gauging your hunger levels four hours later. If you feel famished, try again with a three-quarter-size portion until you reach a level that satisfies you without stuffing.

11

Don't confuse hunger and thirst. I know you've heard this a million times before, but most of us don't drink enough water. Often, we think our body craves food, when we are actually thirsty. I have a friend who hates the advice to drink 2 litres of water so much that she drinks it all in one go – job done! – then feels very bloated. What works for me is to carry a full water bottle in my bag and put it pointedly next to my laptop as I type. Water breaks can then become a displacement activity.

12

Hunger is not always a signal to panic. A day in which you haven't had a couple of spells of feeling slightly peckish is probably a day – sad to say – when you ate too much. I don't mean that you should be getting high on starvation, as happens with some anorexia sufferers, or making a fetish out of going without food. Far from it. Nor am I talking about raging hunger – the kind that, disgracefully, still afflicts millions around the world, even in rich cities such as London. But to feel mildly hungry when you are lucky enough to know that another meal is coming soon is a good thing. 'Hunger is the best sauce' as the saying goes.

13

Ditch the TV dinners (or ration yourself to one a week, maybe on a Saturday night). I know it's hard, especially if you are eating alone, but switch off your phone, at least for ten minutes. When we eat in front of a screen, we seem to eat more and yet also feel less satisfied.

14

Smaller plates – and smaller lunchboxes and smaller wine glasses – really do work (and mean you can minimize wasting food when at home). Eat dinner on side plates or bowls and dessert on saucers. If you spend a week or two weighing everything you eat on digital scales – without actually calorie counting – you start to see how out of kilter our idea of portions has become.

15

Go shopping for your plates at charity chops, jumble sales and antiques markets. Consciously seek out smaller tableware. It shouldn't be hard, and should be much cheaper than buying it new from a department store. I discovered that 28 centimetres has become a normal diameter for a dinner plate, whereas in the 1950s it would have been more like 25 centimetres. We don't *have* to serve ourselves bigger portions just because we are eating off these expanses of china, just as we don't have to drink more when we use large wine glasses. But as it happens, we usually do. Research from Cambridge University in 2015 found that when a wine bar served a standard 175ml measure of wine in larger glasses, people gulped the wine faster because it looked like less.

I have two sets of plates. One set – patterned with birds and flowers – belonged to my grandmother. The other – plain white and minimalist – was given to me when I got married in the late 1990s. It's only recently that I've noticed that when I serve dinner off the large white modern plates, I heap much bigger portions to fill out the space. When we eat from my granny's more modestly sized plates, a smaller helping looks like plenty.

My other invaluable pieces of tableware are ramekins and tiny dipping bowls, the blue and white kind that you can buy from Chinese supermarkets for next to nothing. Often at the end of a meal, I am not really hungry but yearn for something sweet. I find that if I get a dipping bowl and pile it high with whatever I desire – dense chocolate brownies, sticky halva – I feel satisfied, even with a tiny portion. When I first tried this, it felt silly. Could I really be fooled by a plate? Yes. I could. And so could you.

16

Our problem with portions is partly this: no one likes the concept of 'less'. We are conditioned from childhood onwards to yearn for the overflowing glass and the laden table. The inflated portions all around us make it seem positively normal to overeat. As the nutritionist Marion Nestle has remarked: 'It is human nature to eat when presented with food, and to eat more when presented with more food.' We urgently need to invent new models of generosity, until a small portion feels more like kindness than an excessive one. It is not generous for a newsagent to press a 200g bar of chocolate on you when all you wanted was a newspaper. When faced with such excess, don't think 'naughty' or 'shouldn't' but, simply, 'too much'.

17
Revise what counts as a main course. Instead of having a large pizza with a tiny lettuce garnish, have a big plate of roasted peppers and olives with a small pizza on the side. It's still a comforting meal.

18
Try to keep celebration foods for celebrations. One of the many ways our eating has gone wrong is that we find it hard to distinguish celebration foods from everyday ones. This – as usual – is largely the food industry's fault, because foods that were once reserved for high days and holidays are now pushed at us as something to consume whenever we like. This not only encourages us to eat too much, but

ruins the novelty when the real feast comes along. The special pleasure of licking cake mixture from a wooden spoon is not quite so special when your freezer is stocked with cookie-dough ice cream. You may need to make a conscious effort to recalibrate the way you use food to celebrate. Not every happy occasion needs to be marked with a gargantuan cake smothered in sugar. You may find equal joy in a smaller cake, a punnet of cherries and a dance.

19

No one likes waste, but it's time to abandon the idea that it's bad manners to leave food on your plate. Bad manners are to make someone feel ashamed for leaving food on their plate when they are full.

Waste comes in many forms. There is the shocking waste of all the food we throw away. But there is also the human waste of overconsumption, of the people who end up with type 2 diabetes because they habitually consume the wrong food for their body's needs. I have met several people whose family role was to be the 'human dustbin': the person who would eat up all the scraps on everyone's plates to make the rest of the family feel better.

If you are someone who always cleans your plate, it can feel deeply wrong to leave food behind. But in situations – restaurants, let's say – where you can't control the portion you are given, it's really OK.

20

Try to build some generosity into your meals, especially the ones you eat alone. Even as you cut some foods out, add others back in. Breakfast is a good meal to experiment on, because for most of us it is the most heavily ritualized.

I used to start every day with a huge mug of milky coffee, toast, butter, marmalade and juice. Then, I realized that juice was really just sugar. A small glass of orange juice contains twice as much fructose as a whole orange and practically no fibre. To your liver, there is no difference between a glass of juice and a glass of fizzy lemonade laced with high-fructose corn syrup.

So I replaced the juice with a piece of real, whole fruit, with all the benefits of fibre, vitamins and minerals: a juicy pear in autumn, a couple of zesty clementines in winter, a peach or nectarine in summer. This swap was no hardship. I found the whole fruit – with its varied textures and colours – far more enjoyable than the bland sweetness of drinking juice. The children still have juice sometimes, but diluted half and half with water and even they have started to find undiluted juice too sweet.

Then I cut down on sugary marmalade too – though I still have it on the table for old times' sake and may dab it on my final few bites of toast – and switched from milky coffee to black. With the milk gone, I felt there was room in my breakfast for dairy in a different form with a ramekin of yoghurt with toasted nuts or seeds. Now my normal breakfast (give or take the odd plate of eggs or waffles) is: black coffee, whole fruit, yoghurt and nuts, sourdough toast and butter. Sometimes, I have overnight oats or porridge – with various additions – instead of the yoghurt. Even with the juice, the milk and the jam gone, it feels like a fuller, more interesting and varied meal than the breakfasts I ate before.

WHAT TO EAT AND DRINK

You are terrified and beg me to
hold back the thunderbolt? . . .
Calm yourselves; I am going to
describe your diet and show
you that some pleasure still
remains for you, in this world
in which we live to eat.
*Brillat-Savarin, The Physiology
of Taste, 1825*

1

Don't listen to anyone who says they know the one true food that will make you well or ill – including me. I tread warily here. Depending on who's talking, the elixir of life is either seaweed or sauerkraut, quinoa or coffee mixed with butter (strange as it sounds, I did not make this up: search for 'bulletproof coffee'; or rather, don't). There are also many different poisons being touted by various gurus, from gluten to sugar. Some swear that animal fats are good and vegetable fats are bad, and others, equally vehemently, say the opposite. But these prescriptions take no account of the fact that we all react to foods in different ways. We have different microbes, different intolerances, different beliefs about the ethics of food and – perhaps most important of all – different desires.

2

Often, our diverse reactions to food are seen as a problem, but the good news is that we can construct a healthy diet for ourselves in many delicious variations. In 2014 scientists from Yale University studied the evidence to date on which diets were associated with good health. They found that the claims for the superiority of various diets had been exaggerated. The essential tenets of a healthy life are moderate helpings of a variety of real, whole foods, especially plants. But if you can ignore all the crazy clamour of competing diets, it doesn't matter whether we reach this point via a low-carb route or a low-fat one (or vegan or Paleo or just good old-fashioned home cooking).

3

Choose foods that satisfy you rather than the ones you think you ought to eat. The minute we are told that something is diet food, it seems less appealing. When salads were labelled as 'healthy', people found them less satisfying than when the same salads were labelled as 'hearty'.

4

You knew this already, but eating better is never about just one food. My own personal elixir is yoghurt, preferably organic, whole-milk and unsweetened, spooned into small ramekins with a scattering of toasted pumpkin seeds on top. Like other fermented foods, from kimchi to kefir, live yoghurt appears to help digestion. Spooning the mild lactic mixture into my mouth, I feel instantly calm and well (yoghurt contains tryptophan, an amino acid that reduces anxiety). But this is not to say that my yoghurt habit would suit everyone. Maybe you are lactose intolerant, or maybe – like a friend of mine, a slim and sporty man – you just despise the flavour of fermented dairy. Never fear. Yoghurt is not compulsory for good health. Considering how many people – myself included – put our faith in it, the evidence for the overall health benefits of yoghurt remains pretty inconclusive. Do you remember those people in the Caucasus, who supposedly ate yoghurt every day and lived to be a hundred? When an American journalist went to Azerbaijan to interview some of them in the late 1990s, he found that yoghurt wasn't actually very popular among these centenarians, who mostly ate small quantities of vegetables, fruit and sour cheese, while working 'like beasts' in the mountain air. Whatever made them live so long, it wasn't just the yoghurt. It's never just one food.

5

Eat vegetables like a horse and sugar like a bird and everything else in moderation, except for ultra-processed foods, which you should try to eat sparingly and with suspicion, like someone recovering from a nasty bout of stomach flu, for whom each bite is hazardous.

6

We hear a lot about 'superfoods'. The term is used for foods that are supercharged with certain nutrients. Usually, this is a marketing device, trying to get you to hand over your cash for expensive exotica, such as goji berries or wheatgrass. But how many people do you know who actually eat goji berries on a daily basis? The real superfood would be one that you enjoy that also happens to be healthy: crisp, sweet apples, say; or hard-boiled eggs with celery salt for dipping; or warm asparagus with sesame-soy dressing; or deep orange pumpkin soup. A true superfood is affordable enough to eat every day or every week. The more of these superfoods you can build into your personal repertoire, the better you will eat.

7

No food group is forbidden. I'm not going to tell you that all you have to do is give up all carbohydrates and you will never feel hungry again. Because it isn't true. Maybe you'll manage a week or two on a low-carb, high-protein diet; or maybe longer. For prediabetics, there's mounting evidence that low carb diets can help reverse blood sugar problems; but don't take it from me – ask your doctor. For the rest of us, as always, it's complicated. I have friends who felt terrific after giving up all 'sugar' (including bread and alcohol). But life is long and you may not always want to be the person who opts out of what everyone else at the table is eating. The evening may come when you find yourself eating a delicious margherita pizza, bubbling with mozzarella and rich tomato sauce. That's fine. While you're at it, have a glass of red wine on me. Instead of going all-out for a low-carb diet, I personally find it helps to make at least one meal of the day slightly lower in starchy foods than the others. For me, that meal is lunch when I don't want to be weighed down before an afternoon of work. If you don't have much of an appetite in the morning, you might prefer to do it for breakfast. Some are satisfied by a breakfast of nothing more than an avocado and a banana whizzed up with milk and a pinch of cardamom; or toasted hazelnuts with stewed apples and yoghurt; or fried eggs and spinach. Me, I'd add toast. Frankly, if you are sticking to three moderately sized meals of varied food a day, you can have a little carbohydrate at every one without coming to much harm (and if you are an athlete, you can have a little more). For more on specific nutrition for those who exercise a lot, I recommend *Training Food* by Renee McGregor, a dietitian who has worked with British Paralympic athletes.

8

Wean yourself off the ultra-processed products that offer calories without nourishment. What do I mean by 'ultra-processed'? I'm talking about much of what is for sale in a modern supermarket, from sweetened cereals to salty instant noodles and cheese strings. When you see these products, try to stop thinking 'tempting' and start thinking 'inedible'. As of 2014, government statistics show that 23 per cent of calories eaten by the average UK family came from 'foods and drinks high in fat and/or sugar' and our main protein source is 'non-carcase meat and meat products', which basically means cheap processed meat products, from sausages to meat pies. Try to have as few as possible of these items in your kitchen, but don't glamorize them by making them forbidden. For all I know, your well-being may depend on knowing that you can have a sausage roll from time to time. Without cutting these junky foods out altogether, you could tip your diet in a much healthier direction by upping the ratio of non-junk to junk. A bald dinner of meat pie and chips is a very different proposition from a pie with greens.

WHAT TO EAT AND DRINK

9

Avoid foods that make you feel out of control or remorseful. Crisps, for example. As the journalist Michael Moss has documented, food companies work very hard to formulate certain products, especially snack foods, to have exactly the levels of sugar, fat and salt that will provoke you to want more and more once you take a bite. It's generally easier not to have them in the house in the first place.

10

Unsweeten your palate. I don't happen to believe that sugar fully deserves the opprobrium currently being heaped upon it. Apart from anything else, most of us associate sweet things with happy times, so when we hear someone reviling these treats, it can make us feel personally attacked. There are worse things in this life than a slice of treacle tart and clotted cream. But when it reaches the stage where sugar is present in 80 per cent of all items for sale in the supermarket – including pasta sauce, chicken ready-meals and bread – it's time to take our sweet tooth down several notches. Sugar was never meant to be a staple food. Biologists have found that if we consistently eat less sugar, it changes our sense of sweetness. If we could only take a fortnight's holiday from sugar, we might return to it less fondly. That includes agave, maple syrup, manuka honey and all those other posh sweeteners that pretend not to be anything as vulgar as 'sugar' but are in fact metabolized by the body in exactly the same way as the white granulated stuff in your sugar bowl. When your palate changes away from intense sweetness, you start to enjoy foods you never considered to be sweet before. The day may come when you notice the sweetness in a whole cob of buttery corn at the height of summer; or a dish of fennel cooked long and slow until it is toffee brown.

SIX WAYS TO UNSWEETEN YOUR PALATE

If you wish you didn't have such a sweet tooth, consider going cold turkey on sweetened drinks. This includes sugary tea, and – sorry! – those lovely organic elderflowers as well as diet drinks. I know it seems as if artificially sweetened drinks will help you to eat less (I've been there) but as long as you are coating your mouth in sweetness several times a day, your palate will be skewed towards sugar. There's also evidence that, annoyingly, frequent consumption of diet drinks is associated with higher levels of type 2 diabetes and weight gain, for reasons that aren't entirely clear.

If you were using these drinks as a crutch to see you through the hungry hour before dinner or to avoid alcohol, replace some of them with fizzy water and a squeeze of lime (purists would say this is still bad for your teeth, so don't be a purist). If you find this rule too strict, build a couple of sweet drinks into your week, but treat them with ceremony and sip slowly, as you might a gin and tonic (which is also sugar, by the way).

If you don't want to give up juice, cut it half-and-half with water. Gradually work your way down to three-quarters water to a quarter juice. The undiluted stuff should now taste horribly intense.

When baking, cut the amount of sugar in the recipe down by a third. This will affect the texture slightly, but with most recipes (except for those cookies that need the sugar to crisp up), it works perfectly fine.

Buy porridge oats, cereals, yoghurt and similar in unsweetened form and add any sweet element – such as fruit or honey – yourself. The ready-sweetened versions are all crazily over-sugared. I never thought I could enjoy plain yoghurt without sizeable dollops of honey or brown sugar and was startled when my palate changed enough for me to notice the sweetness in the plain milky yoghurt itself.

Try to rely as little as possible on supermarket ready-meals, which can be astonishingly sugary even when supposedly savoury.

11

Cultivate a taste for bitterness, from bitter green leaves to artichokes and lemon zest. A penchant for bitterness has many advantages. For one thing it makes you less susceptible to the endless sugar that greets us in every shop. The bitterness has increasingly been bred out of fruits and vegetables – even grapefruits. A quest for bitter will help you to adjust your palate away from the ubiquitous sweetness of our food supply. Bitterness also seems to help us to eat less. New research presented at the European Obesity Summit in June 2016 suggested that ingesting certain bitter plant extracts may trigger the feeling of fullness in the gut, acting as a kind of 'bitter brake' on our eating. This makes sense. I certainly find that the lingering pucker of bitterness in the mouth means that, much as I love bitter substances, from espresso to Seville oranges, I can't consume very much of them.

12

Don't be scared of fat. Some variations of a high-fat diet, it now turns out, are probably less fattening and damaging to health than all those low-fat diets high in refined carbohydrates. A review of sixty-five studies found no link between consumption of saturated fats and heart disease. Not all fat is the same. Synthetic trans fats – which, luckily, are being phased out of most manufactured foods – have no benefits, and seem to contribute to heart disease. Refined vegetable oils – such as sunflower and peanut oil – may also be slightly less healthy than we once thought, because they are high in omega-6 fats, which modern Western diets already contain too much of (my own feeling is that a little sunflower oil in a stir-fry is no disaster, but you can make up your own mind). Many people now consider virgin coconut oil to be a panacea, but if you can't afford £8 for a jar, don't despair. There is a wealth of other good fats to choose: from butter to lard, from grapeseed to walnut oil. If in doubt, choose extra virgin olive oil, the health benefits of which have never been disputed and which, just as importantly, is delicious. Nutrition aside, fat is filling and it carries flavour like nothing else and therefore helps you to eat smaller portions. Zero-fat yoghurt gives me no more satisfaction than gruel. I end up eating more of it, searching for a bite that actually tastes of something.

13

As you change your diet, pay more attention to the foods you are adding than the ones you are cutting out. Professor Tim Lang of City University, London, advocates eating as many as seven or even nine vegetables and fruits a day rather than the official UK advice of five a day. Lang – who grows his own vegetables – follows the nine-a-day advice himself. He finds that apart from the copious health benefits of the fruits and vegetables themselves – the fibre, the vitamins, the anti-carcinogenic properties – in these quantities it leaves him too full to eat very large amounts of anything else, including junk food.

14

Save your nourishment for food rather than drink, wherever possible. It's easy to take in far more energy than you intended in the form of drinks, mindlessly consumed (calories in a grande latte or a 250ml fruit smoothie: around 200). Over the course of a day, a coffee drinker whose default is cappuccino or latte can easily drink as much as 750ml milk without really thinking about it. Switching to black or white

Americanos or tea is a fairly painless swap. This is not to say that you should never have a drink containing calories (a large glass of Rioja sits next to me right now as I write. Cheers!). But if you are going to have these drinks, you might as well be aware what you are doing. Regard anything other than water, tea and black coffee more as snacks than drinks. Because black coffee is my default now, on the occasions when I do have a flat white – preferably one of those hipster ones with latte art on top – I appreciate how rich and filling it is.

15

A word about fruit. Diet experts are increasingly divided on how much fruit we should eat. Some nutritionists say that fruits – especially very sweet types such as mangoes, bananas, grapes and pineapple – are really 'just' sugar and no better for your body than marshmallow fluff. But the official advice is still to eat *more* fruit, as part of your five-a-day. Supermarkets push those rainbow tubs of 'fresh' fruit salad (the cut fruit is doused in various chemical dips to stop it browning, as food campaigner Joanna Blythman has exposed) as a healthy option: get two of your five-a-day in a single portion!

I say both the anti-fruiters and the pro-fruiters are wrong. Yes, fruit can be sweet, but that is exactly why it is lovely to eat. No one *needs* to eat a passion fruit. You shouldn't feel obliged to swallow fruit because it is good for you – although the fibre and vitamins in an apple make it far better for you than other sweet foods. Fruit is a treat, to be savoured. It is absurd that anyone should eat a handful of ripe June cherries and congratulate themselves on a job done. Stop seeing ripe fruit as something you either *should* or *shouldn't* eat, and start seeing it as one of life's everyday luxuries, to be eaten more sparingly than vegetables, but still to be eaten.

Our ancestors had the right idea about fruit. They saw it as something heady and tempting. It was dessert, not duty. In seventeenth-century France there was a mania for melon, which one poet (Saint-Amant) described as 'a new and pure ambrosia', better than the kisses of a mistress. I wouldn't go quite that far, but I do regard a ripe orange melon as one of the most seductive things the table has to offer.

Instant melon sorbet

If you have a food processor, you can make the most luscious instant 'sorbets' from overripe fruit. No ice cream maker required. Any soft fruit – from bananas to nectarines – can be washed or peeled, chopped and frozen, ready to be whizzed into a gelato-textured treat. It's a good solution to the perennial problem of brown bananas. But my favourite is this elegant one with heady orange melon, just the thing to calm frazzled nerves on a heavy August day. Some might call this divine coral-coloured ice a 'guilt-free dessert'. I call it a delight.

Makes 4–6 portions
1 whole melon, preferably cantaloupe or Charentais
3 tablespoons apple juice
juice of a lime
2 tablespoons icing sugar

The day before you want to eat it, peel and chop the melon into largeish chunks, discarding the seeds. Put it in a plastic box with a lid in the freezer. It can be kept in the freezer for up to three months so you can make sorbet whenever the mood takes you.

Take the melon from the freezer. If the pieces are totally solid and joined together, sit the box in a dish of hot kettle-water for 30 seconds. Put it in the food processor with all the other ingredients. Process for 2–3 minutes, until you have a smooth, pinky-golden ice cream with a soft consistency. If it just won't go smooth, add more apple juice, half a spoonful at a time. Pile into glasses and eat at once. If you don't have enough people round the table to eat it up in a sitting, any leftovers can be refrozen for up to a week, but the texture will harden.

16

Eat like a vegetarian, without necessarily being one. The amount of animal products we eat in rich countries like Britain and the US is historically unprecedented. This is having a disastrous impact on the environment (not to mention on animals). Meat production, especially beef, generates more climate-warming emissions than cars. What we don't talk about so much – maybe because we've been conditioned to think of 'protein' as a wonder food – is the human cost of meat eating. Large studies in Britain and Germany have found that non-meat eaters are 40 per cent less likely to develop certain cancers than regular carnivores. Contrary to what the low-carbists may say, high meat consumption has also been linked to weight gain in a study of 400,000 Europeans. You may not choose to give up meat completely. I am certainly no vegan. Having experimented with excluding it altogether, I personally feel better with a little meat in my diet, whether it's for the B vitamins, the iron or the joy of roast chicken. But the operative word is little.

17

Eat soup.

A reason? Let me count them. It's delicious (how often do you ever meet someone who says they hate soup?). It can be made quickly from the humblest ingredients. It's healthy and infinitely varied. It's an easy way to eat vegetables. And it makes us feel loved. Soup is like salad, but without the atmosphere of obligation.

Soup – in all its varieties, from broth to chowder – seems to have a remarkable ability to fill us up, even when it contains few calories. Scientists at Purdue University found that when people drank a glass of apple juice, it did not make them full. But when they were given the same juice heated up and presented as 'apple soup', they were still full an hour later. It is the *idea* of soup that makes us full, as much as anything. Soup can nurture and nourish you like nothing else. It's what our mothers gave us when we were ill. It's health food and comfort in a single bowl.

Lentil soup for every season

Everyone should know how to make lentil soup. It's about the cheapest meal you can make, it's full of protein and fibre and can be varied infinitely, depending on mood and season and what you happen to have in the cupboard. It is good spiced or unspiced. Best of all, it makes you feel properly *fed*. If you fear that lentils will taste austere, start with red lentils, which are the quickest to cook and can be whizzed to a creamy purée that could almost be pumpkin soup, if you didn't know different.

Serves 4

2 tablespoons olive oil

1 onion, peeled and finely chopped

2 sticks celery, finely chopped

2 carrots, peeled and finely chopped

2 cloves garlic, peeled and chopped

1 teaspoon Maldon sea salt

250g red lentils

1 bay leaf

1 litre unsalted stock or water

a squeeze of lemon

optional garnish: a few leaves of Savoy cabbage,
    shredded

1 tablespoon olive oil

a pinch of Maldon sea salt and a pinch of sugar

Heat the oil in a casserole dish and soften the onion, celery, carrot and garlic for a few minutes. Add the salt and stir for a minute more. Rinse the lentils in a sieve under running water and add them along with the bay leaf and stock or water and simmer for 15 minutes or until the lentils have swollen into a creamy mass. If any scum appears, just remove it with a ladle. Remove the bay leaf. If it's too thick, add an extra 200ml water. You can eat it as it is or whizz until very smooth with a hand-held blender. Season to taste with lemon juice. If you want to make the optional garnish, fry the cabbage leaves in the oil until slightly crispy with the pinches of salt and sugar. Serve the soup with a few crispy-fried leaves in each bowl.

LENTIL SOUP VARIATIONS

Fennel and butternut squash: replace the carrot and celery with a small bulb of fennel and a small butternut squash (about 400g peeled weight), both chopped. Add a little chopped rosemary as the vegetables soften. I might add a spoonful or two of cream or crème fraîche at the end and the zest as well as the juice of the lemon, plus some chopped flat-leaf parsley. And Parmesan.

Spiced green lentils and spinach: add a teaspoon each of ground cumin and ground coriander as the vegetables soften. Replace the red lentils with green or brown lentils and cook for 20–30 minutes instead of 15, topping up with water if it dries out. Shred 200g washed spinach and stir it in at the end, until wilted. Eat with yoghurt and a sprinkle of cayenne.

Puy lentil, pasta and chorizo: add 100g chopped chorizo, along with the onion and celery (no carrot for this one) and 2 large chopped tomatoes along with the lentils. Use Puy lentils instead of red and cook for 20–30 minutes instead of 15. Ten minutes before the end of the cooking time, boil some soup pasta according to the packet instructions and add some to each bowl. You can cook the pasta in the soup if you prefer, but any leftovers will go soggy.

18

I promised I wouldn't give you dietary advice. But if I could ask you to do one simple thing, it would be this: consider taking a holiday from sandwiches, if not for a lifetime, at least for a month.

What's wrong with sandwiches? In theory, nothing. A good sandwich followed by a piece of fruit can be one of the great meals, and a balanced and filling one too: good rye bread piled with buffalo mozzarella, salt, tomatoes and basil; a porchetta roll (Italian roast pork) heady with rosemary and fried courgettes; smoked trout, horseradish, crème fraîche and watercress on sourdough. But how often – be honest – are the sandwiches you eat anything like this? When I stopped eating sandwiches as my basic lunch a couple of years ago, I lost half a stone without trying. A sandwich habit is one of the ways that – even if you are not unhappy about eating, or a binge eater – added weight can creep up on you.

Most sandwiches in the shops are made with bad sliced bread – 'multigrain' or not – a lot of industrial mayonnaise and contain few if any vegetables. Most 'home-made' sandwiches are made from the same poor quality bread and processed meat or cheese. Nearly a quarter of British people eat a ham sandwich for lunch *every weekday*, according to a survey from 2012; and a further 22 per cent eat a cheese sandwich.

To make matters worse, sandwiches are often eaten in the form of a supermarket 'meal deal' with a packet of crisps and a sweetened drink, which you pick up automatically because it would feel foolish to turn down the opportunity. A £3 supermarket 'meal deal' of chicken sandwich, small packet of crisps and fizzy drink can easily contain more than 700 calories, 30g of sugar and not a single piece of greenery or fruitery.

This is exactly why I'm suggesting you give them up, at least for a while. Because sandwiches are the default midday meal for most of us, the act of relinquishing them is the single easiest thing you can do right now to recalibrate the way you eat for the better without going on a diet. If lunch isn't a sandwich, what is it? You'll be forced to think far more carefully about what you eat and the chances are that you will consume far more vegetables (unless you swap your sandwich for a Cornish pasty, in which case all bets are off). You may – see above – decide that the best of all lunches is soup. You may start eating hearty dishes of grains and greens; flasks of warming stew; boxes of chickpeas or lentils dressed with oil, herbs and caramelized walnuts and preserved lemons. When you are not trapped by the sandwich mindset, you start to see that lunch could be last night's pilaf thriftily reclaimed as a rice salad with herbs and nuts and olives.

Pausing your sandwich habit will free you up to widen your food horizons. When you are not limited by the format of something between two slices of bread, you can eat anything. In short, you can eat food, in all its varied glory.

After a month, you are free to return to sandwiches, or not, as you wish. But I guarantee you the old habitual nondescript sandwich won't seem quite as appetizing. You notice a certain dampness about the bread, a feeling of heaviness at your desk an hour after you have eaten. Your concept both of filling and of bread should now have altered. There still may be mornings when – sad or hung over – only a bacon butty with ketchup will do.

But you may also find yourself doing crazy things like making sandwiches from garlicky pak choi and tofu stuffed into flatbread; or roasted aubergines with halloumi. Something will have shifted in the way you see lunch. Given how many lunches there are in a life, this is not a small thing.

19

A word about bread. Ever more people are shunning bread and turning to gluten-free diets. Bread sales in Britain are in long-term decline (except for the bread in sandwiches). This is no tragedy, given that almost everything sold as 'bread' is of terrible quality, 'multigrain' or no. It is neither proved nor fermented but hastily made in a factory by the Chorleywood process using lots of additives and processing aids (see realbreadcampaign.org for more on what's wrong with industrial bread). But real, hefty properly made bread – the kind with a sweet crumb and a toothsome crust – definitely has a place in a balanced diet. Without a staple food such as bread, our eating can start to feel unmoored. Many people who think they can't tolerate bread are actually reacting to the large quantities of yeast in industrial bread and would do fine with real, slow-fermented breads.

It's striking that in Denmark, where they eat large quantities of old-fashioned dense, dark rye bread, child obesity rates are much lower than in Britain. It can be hard to lay your hands on real bread here, especially if you can't always afford the artisanal kind that costs £4 a loaf. The Village Bakery rye bread is the cheapest good bread I've found in supermarkets. Or consider baking your own. Making sourdough can be a form of therapy. I make my dough in the bread-maker to save time, then shape it by hand.

20

Don't eat as if you have a food intolerance unless you actually have one. Humans thrive best on nourishing and varied fuel. Your body gets no goodness from the foods that you cut out, only from the ones that you put in your mouth, chew and digest.

COOKING

Anyone who likes to eat, can
soon learn to cook well.
Jane Grigson, Good Things, 1970

1

Most people eat much better when most of what they eat is home-cooked. Cooking is the best way to take control of your own nourishment. But this principle only works if you make at least a few things other than cupcakes. Judging from the cookware sections of modern shops, people mainly use their kitchens for cake and cappuccino. When I was a compulsive eater, I cooked all the time, but it didn't make me eat well. My idea of a fun afternoon was a few hours with wooden spoons and whisks, baking brioche and macaroons from scratch, wolfing down the fruits of my labours hot from the oven in a remorseful haze. I knew how to make nut brittle and fudge and coffee buttercream – impressive cooking skills but not ones that necessarily did my well-being much good. It pains me to say it, because cooking gives rhythm and meaning to my days, but some non-cooks actually eat better than cooks. If you have a balanced relationship with food, you can sustain yourself pretty well with such things as ripe cheese, tomatoes, olives, bread and fruit. For cooking to become the solution to our diet crisis, we first have to learn how to adjust our responses to food so that we *want* to cook different things.

2

Cook with a view to changing your tastes. Tempt yourself with new dishes, and comfort yourself with familiar ones.

3

The point of cooking is not to impress but to *feed*. Unless you are a chef, the kind of cooking that really matters most is not the dinner party masterpiece or the epic Christmas dinner. Cookbook author Anna Jones says it's what we cook on a Tuesday or Wednesday that really makes the difference. I agree. When you've got enough recipes in your head to rustle up a warming one-pot meal on a rainy midweek evening, you are winning.

4

If you are trying to lose weight, don't feel you must only use 'diet' recipes or 'clean eating' ones, which can often feel dreary and faddy. It's much better to learn how to cook from a cookbook that puts flavours first, because you are more likely to make the recipes a regular part of your life. A recipe for a dietetically perfect goji berry and quinoa salad that you make only once is far less useful than a trusty formula for a stir-fry that you return to time and again. If you cook a variety of dishes, and concentrate on meals involving vegetables, you can't go far wrong. And stick to the advised portion sizes, although you'll soon discover that the meaning of 'serves 4' can vary wildly; tweak the quantities accordingly. If you always use the same, smallish plates, as suggested above, you should be fine.

5

Try to ignore all the persistent messages – many of them put out by companies trying to sell you takeaways or ready-meals – about how you just don't have time to cook and must therefore buy in. Feeding yourself well through cooking is something that's always worth investing time in, even if you don't quite manage it every day.

6

No spa treatment is as relaxing as the calm that descends when yolk meets oil under a whisk and emulsifies into a shining lake of mayonnaise.

7

When you cook, put your faith in cuisines more than in nutrients. Traditional cuisines across the world – from Greece to Italy to China – were founded on a strong sense of balance, with norms about which foods go together, and how much one should eat at different times of day. Much cooking now, however, is nothing like this, whether it's based on so-called 'healthy' ingredients or not.

8

Treat greens as lavishly and thoughtfully as if they were chocolate. Don't think you always have to steam them to minimize the calories (although simple steamed vegetables can be excellent if you start with good vegetables and get the timing right). If you want yourself to love vegetables more, vary your cooking methods. Mashed potato lovers might convert themselves to celeriac or parsnip by mashing them with butter. Frying or roasting is often a good entry point for vegetables you think you dislike, because heat plus oil brings out the sweetness. Take a cabbage, cut it into wedges, anoint it with a little olive oil and nigella seeds and blister it on a tray in a hot oven until the edges are brown and crispy. Sprinkle with salt. It then becomes something nutty and sweet.

9

Use spice. Spices have the power to make us desire food that might otherwise seem unexciting. I find it odd that governments, despite trying so hard to persuade us to eat more of certain foods and less of others, have not tapped this potential. The right spices can help you wean yourself away from the intense flavours of processed food. A teaspoon of cinnamon mixed with a pinch of cardamom sprinkled on porridge is so heady that you can almost do without sugar. Almost.

10

No one is too busy to cook. If you can make time in your day to brush your teeth and check your Twitter feed, you can find the time to cook. You may have to be inventive about when that time is, though. I'm convinced that one of the main reasons more people don't cook is not because we are lazy but because the usual slot for cooking – between five and seven in the evening – is crowded with so many other urgent claims on our attention, from last-minute work queries to ferrying small people to after-school activities. On extra-frantic days, I sometimes cook both lunch and dinner in a thirty-minute window after breakfast. It can be done, and when you get in the swing of it, it isn't hard to make a big bowl of rice noodles with vegetables and cashews for everyone's lunchboxes (rice noodles cook in three minutes or less) at the same time as making something like a comforting frittata of red onions, sweet potatoes and herbs, ready for supper.

If that sounds too manic (and I see your point), you might find that cooking in the evening, *after* you've eaten, is another possibility. This way, you can stir and chop without the stress of a deadline and you don't need to worry so much if something takes an hour or more to cook. It's a wonderful treat waking up the next day and finding something in the fridge – a Greek spinach pie, a moussaka, a spicy tagine – that you thoughtfully prepared earlier. It's as if the fairies have left it. Other times, though, you may prefer to cook something immediately, on the hoof. Simple cooking isn't as easy as pie – it's much easier. If you have a bag of frozen peas, and a pan, you can make soup. Add a large pinch of salt, a couple of spring onions if you have them (ditto a stick or two of celery), cover with boiling water from a kettle and cook for 10 minutes. Blitz with a hand-held blender, adding crème fraîche or olive oil as you go, and maybe a handful of mint or tarragon. Or – on one of those nights when you have rushed back from somewhere and feel as if you hardly have time to breathe, never mind cook – think of chopping a red pepper, and softening in oil for a couple of minutes. Add a clove of garlic and two eggs and stir. In under a minute, you have a healthy feast for one, to eat with sourdough toast.

11

Instead of buying convenience foods, invest in convenience kitchen equipment that makes the task of cooking fresh meals every day less of a grind. Exactly what form this equipment will take depends on your temperament, household size and routines. One of the reasons that many people don't eat as many vegetables as they might is because they think that prepping them is a drag. Those people do not own sharp knives or a salad spinner. Everyone needs a sharp knife, an ergonomic vegetable peeler and a good chopping board. One really sharp knife is better than ten blunt ones, so I personally would not now wish to cook without a good knife sharpener (mine is electric). Another huge time-saver, and a cheap one, is a hand-held blender (for blitzing everything from smooth soups to hummus, home-made pestos and green coriander chutney).

Depending on your routines and how impatient you are (I am *very*), you might want to get either a slow cooker or a pressure cooker. I resisted a pressure cooker for years, then got one, and became a total convert (thanks in part to *The Pressure Cooker Cookbook* by Catherine Phipps). Suddenly I could make risotto or soup in ten minutes with no stirring and casseroles that were better than the ones I used to make that took five hours in the oven. The pressure cooker transformed my cooking repertoire, because dishes that I'd once dismissed as too much effort for midweek suppers were suddenly doable. A case in point is this fragrant sort-of Vietnamese chicken soup, which tastes as deeply savoury as if someone has been tending it with a ladle half the day but is actually ready in thirty minutes of minimal work. You can still make it in a normal pan – I'll explain how below – but you'll just have to wait a bit longer.

My pho

I think of chicken pho as the essence of not-diet food,
by which I mean it makes me feel energized and well
but not remotely deprived. I've never been to
Vietnam, so can't claim authenticity. But it does taste
authentically good: rich salty noodle broth scented
with star anise, with the zing of lime and mint. 'This
tastes like it could cure flu,' said my daughter last
time I made it.

Serves 6
1 tablespoon oil (whatever you have)
2 onions, peeled and quartered
1 thumb of ginger, sliced
4 whole free-range chicken legs or 1 small whole free-
    range chicken or guinea-fowl cut into four
1 dessertspoon Maldon sea salt
1 dessertspoon brown sugar
3 whole star anise
1 cinnamon stick, snapped in half
1 dessertspoon coriander seeds
1.75 litres water
400g thin rice noodles
fresh mint and coriander leaves (if you only want to
    buy one lot of herbs, go for mint)

1 fresh chilli

3 yellow courgettes, halved and very thinly sliced
    (beansprouts are more traditional so use them if
    you prefer – 200g – but I like the crunch and
    colour of courgettes)

2 limes, cut into wedges

soy sauce or fish sauce

chilli sauce (Sriracha)

Heat the oil in the pressure cooker and cook the onion and ginger over a high heat until slightly charred. Add the chicken, salt, sugar, all the spices and the water. Close the lid and bring to high pressure over a high heat. Turn the heat down and cook for 20 minutes.

If you don't have a pressure cooker, proceed exactly the same in a big saucepan, bring to simmering, skim off the scum and simmer very gently for 1 to 1½ hours (check if the chicken is falling off the bone).

Either way, while it is cooking, prepare all the accompaniments: soak the noodles in hot water following the instructions on the packet, then rinse and drain; wash the herbs, chop the chilli. Fast-release the pressure cooker by pouring cold water over the lid until the pressure goes down completely.

Be extremely careful not to open the lid until the pressure has released; being scalded by hot stock is not fun.

Strain the stock into another pan. As soon as the chicken is cool enough to handle, shred the meat – which should be very soft – from the bone, avoiding the skin. Skim any scum and the top layer of fat from the stock, but leave some shimmering beads of fat. This is schmaltz and it carries flavour.

To serve the pho, put some rice noodles and chicken in each bowl, pour over hot stock (it should now smell heavenly) and add herbs and courgettes or beansprouts on top. My fussy 7-year-old likes it with just noodles, chicken and broth, with vegetables on the side. Let people add their own lime juice and soy or fish sauce to taste, plus fresh chilli and/or chilli sauce, depending on how hot you like it.

12

If you hate prepping vegetables, do enough at a time to last you for a few days and put them in a Ziploc bag in the salad compartment in the fridge.

13

If you only learn how to cook one thing, let that thing be eggs.

Eggs are nutrient-packed, affordable, high in protein and the source of countless dinners that are on the table in under ten minutes. I am amazed by how many people still don't know how to boil an egg. Here's how I do it (for soft-boiled eggs with soldiers, for a solitary lunch). Boil a kettle and pour it into a small saucepan over medium heat. Lower in two large eggs using a slotted spoon, turn the heat down to simmer and boil for six minutes. While they are boiling, make toast and steam some asparagus or tenderstem broccoli. Dip alternate bites of buttered toast and green spears into the runny golden yolk.

14

Comfort eating isn't necessarily a bad thing. Sometimes it's the only kind of eating we are capable of. Everyone should know how to cook at least a few things that console them deep to their core. We all have days that defeat us. It helps if you know you can make yourself a bowlful of something warm and undemanding at short notice. After Joan Didion's husband died, as she recounts in *The Year of Magical Thinking*, a friend brought round a quart of scallion and ginger congee (rice porridge) from Chinatown. 'Congee was all I could eat,' writes Didion.

The trouble with the 'comfort food' that most people eat is that it doesn't truly comfort us. We eat too much of it and then feel awful, from additives and guilt. Real comfort food, by contrast, is bolstering and provokes none of that morning-after regret. In 1989 San Francisco suffered an earthquake, and in the aftermath restaurant takings went down as people felt nervous to go out. The Zuni Café, run by the great chef Judy Rodgers, stayed in business during those difficult months by selling many more orders than usual of their famous $5 polenta: yellow grainy comfort in a bowl. We should all build up our own repertoire of foods to cook and eat when the earthquake hits. These are two of mine.

TWO COMFORT FOODS, ONE SAVOURY, ONE SWEET

Each serves 1

Mushroom polenta

The best polenta is made from coarse cornmeal and takes up to forty-five minutes to cook with continuous stirring, but on the days I feel in need of polenta – usually after I've been to the gym – I don't have the energy. Quick-cook is a fine compromise, if you add enough salt and butter.

Boil a kettle. Put 80g quick-cook polenta in a pan. Pour over 200ml water from the kettle, add a big pinch of salt and stir continuously for 2–3 minutes or until thick and porridgy. Add more water as you go if it needs it. Add a little piece of butter and taste for salt. Meanwhile, cook 100g sliced mushrooms – any kind – in a big lump of butter with a big pinch of salt until reduced in size, browned and savoury. Pour the buttery mushrooms over the polenta in a bowl. Add a grating of nutmeg and a squeeze of lemon and eat with a spoon. Don't be tempted to add parsley, because it would interrupt the comforting texture.

Tahini and black sesame porridge

Tahini – aka sesame paste – adds a magical richness to porridge. The other key ingredient here is a piece of vanilla pod which makes the porridge taste luxurious. Expensive, I know, but you only need a small fragment. Put 125ml porridge oats in a pan with a small piece of vanilla pod and 375ml water or milk and water mixed. Add a pinch of salt. Bring to the boil and simmer, stirring frequently, for 3 minutes or until thick. Pour into a bowl and stir in a heaped teaspoon of tahini. Sprinkle over black sesame seeds and a drizzle of honey. I might have a sliced fresh fig with this.

15

When learning how to cook, focus on the dishes you actually want yourself to eat. We are not 1950s housewives. It's far more useful to know how to make one really delicious stew than any number of elaborate pies. Cooks – especially women – often feel judged on their ability to turn out 'perfect' pastry. But goodish pastry – whether filo or puff – is easily bought. What you can't buy – at least, not cheaply – is a wholesome, heart-warming family soup or stew.

Basil and lemon stew

This is somewhere between minestrone and Greek avgolemono in flavour, but quicker than either. I find it both comforting and uplifting. It's the sort of thing you can make when you arrive home on a Saturday lunchtime with almost no time to cook and you crave something less stodgy than a cheese sandwich (though, come to think of it, grilled cheese on toast would go well alongside, if you are hungry).

Serves 4, maybe with leftovers
2 tablespoons olive oil
1 large onion, red or brown, peeled and chopped
2 red or orange peppers
4 large carrots
2 cloves garlic
1 teaspoon Maldon sea salt
300g waxy potatoes
1 x 400g can cannellini beans
1 litre water or unsalted stock
1 lemon
80ml whole-milk yoghurt (not Greek)
more yoghurt to serve
1 bunch basil

I make this in a pressure cooker to save time, but it's fine in a normal saucepan too. I find this kind of soup easiest if you prep the vegetables in stages. In the pressure cooker or pan, heat the oil and soften the onion. While this is happening, wash and chop the peppers and add to the pan, giving it a good stir now and then. Now, peel and chop the carrots and add them. Peel and chop the garlic and add that too, along with the salt which will help stop the vegetables from browning. Peel and chop the potatoes and add them, along with the drained beans. Stir and add the water or stock. If using a pressure cooker, bring to high pressure for 2 minutes and fast release. If using a normal pan, bring to a simmer, put on the lid, turn the heat down and cook for 10 minutes or until the potatoes are tender. Either way, season with the zest and juice of the lemon. Check for salt and slowly stir in the yoghurt, off the heat so that it doesn't curdle. Serve with more yoghurt and a big handful of fresh basil in each bowl.

16

Take nourishment from the cooking process as well as from the end result. Feel the fluffy soft insides of a broad bean pod. Smell the garlic as it sizzles in oil. Hear how the risotto rice seems to sigh with relief when you feed it the first ladleful of wine and stock.

17

Healthy cooking doesn't have to be expensive. Diet books sometimes give the impression that you can't eat well unless you have the cash for oceans of maple syrup and obscure ingredients such as bee pollen and yuzu juice. Luckily, it isn't true. If you can ignore what is trendy, there are plenty of dishes that are both thrifty and good for you. I love making softly spiced pilaffs from whatever vegetables are left in the fridge at the end of the week, fluffed up at the end with butter and flaked almonds, if I have any. This works especially well with sweet root vegetables. Another cheap-as-chips dinner could be bubble and squeak made with spring greens – spring greens are one of the last great bargains, like kale without the pretension – and a poached egg. Or consider the gratin. Few dinners are cheaper, or more delicious than a vegetable gratin, cooked slowly in the oven in a mixture of stock and cream: you can make a glorious purple one from beetroot and potatoes (a Lucas Hollweg idea) that only needs a cucumber salad with feta and tarragon to become a feast.

You can also save a fortune by not overstocking your cupboards. I used to have four or five different vinegars on the go at any given time. Now, I find that just one (at the moment, I like apple cider vinegar) will answer pretty much every need.

18

Nothing you can buy – not gym membership, not hot rock massage – will give you quite the same degree of health and pleasure as good ingredients to cook with. View it as preventive medicine, of the most delicious kind. Most of us could afford to spend more on food than we do. I'm not saying that *everyone* could; it's a scandal that there are still households in modern Britain where parents need to go without lunch to see their children eat. But the majority of families could spend a little more on food if they chose to. Historically, we have never spent such a low percentage of our income on food. Based on figures from *The Economist* in 2013, the British now spend on average under 10 per cent of household income on food, compared to Japan where they spend 15 per cent (and where rates of diet-related ill health are much lower). It's a sign of misplaced priorities. By spending so little on cooking, we are effectively saying it doesn't matter. In our busy lives, it's easy to give cooking second billing to other activities: homework, after-school activities, Instagram. The problem is partly that the prevalence of ready-meals gives us false ideas about how much food should cost. A real home-made fish pie, cooked from scratch, will cost far more than a 99p frozen one; but it will also do you a great deal more good, both in the short run and the long run.

19

Overcome your aversion to cooking with fish. Compared to meat, we consume vanishingly small quantities of fish, yet it's one of the healthiest foods you can eat, especially small oily fish such as herring and mackerel. I suspect we have two problems with fresh fish. 1) We don't like eating it. 2) We don't like cooking it. You can avoid the cooking part by cultivating a taste for canned sardines or smoked mackerel, both very cheap sources of protein and omega-3, and delicious on toast with plenty of lemon. But as it happens, fish is easier to cook than meat. Take fresh sardines. Just rub the whole gutted sardines (two per person) with oil, add salt and grill for four minutes a side under a hot grill (check after three minutes). Eat with oregano, lemon and a green salad and imagine you are on holiday in Greece.

Or make white fish in a parcel with radish, leek and thyme: a complete meal, as simple as wrapping a birthday present. The flavours concentrate inside the paper, without any fishy cooking smells. Per person, take one roughly 125g fillet of white fish (cod, haddock, pollock, anything sustainable and fresh, defrosted if frozen) and two large sheets of baking parchment (30 by 40cm, layered one on top of the other). Put a teaspoon of extra virgin olive oil on the top layer of paper, add the fish and season well with salt. Thinly slice a leek, cut a carrot into thin batons and put on top of the fish with a crushed clove of garlic, the leaves from a sprig or two of thyme, a tablespoon of dry vermouth or white wine, five pink radishes, sliced, and another teaspoon of oil. Hold the two longer ends of the paper together and fold over several times. Carefully fold the sides in, until it feels secure. Make as many parcels as there are people to feed. You can keep the parcels in the fridge until you are ready to eat. Preheat the oven to 200°C. Bake on a tray for twenty minutes. The parcel should puff up with the steam. Let it rest for five minutes. When you open it, be careful not to lose the juices.

Devour by itself, or with waxy new potatoes. The vegetables can be varied in countless ways. *Red pepper and olive*: 2 teaspoons olive oil, 1 tablespoon dry vermouth, ½ red pepper, ½ fennel bulb, 1 garlic clove, 1 tablespoon chopped flat-leaf parsley, zest of half a lemon and a handful of olives. *Ginger and mushroom*: 50g sliced mushrooms, briefly sautéed in 1 teaspoon oil, a knob of butter, 1 tablespoon dry sherry, 2 teaspoons chopped pickled ginger, ½ sliced red onion, 1 whole star anise, 1 dessertspoon soy sauce, and chives at the end.

20

A taste for home-cooked food can be like a life-jacket, protecting you from the worst excesses of the obesogenic world we now inhabit. Once you are hooked on home-cooked flavours, a gloopy, salty ready-meal no longer appeals. You see the greasy meatball sandwich and it no longer speaks to you, because you know it is nothing compared to the meatballs you can make in the warmth of your own kitchen.

CHILDREN

Don't urge, don't coax, don't
force, don't bribe.
Hazel Kepler and Elizabeth Hesser,
Food for Little People, 1950

1

There is no single 'right' way to feed children and close your ears to anyone who pretends different. What works for one family may not work for another. You can make plenty of mistakes (I did with my three and as a food writer I should have known better) and still end up with kids who eventually eat a pretty OK diet.

2

Most parents let their kids choose which breakfast cereal to buy but tell them which vegetables to eat. It should be the other way round.

3

Nothing a parent tells a child about food will ever be as powerful as the way they see you behave at the table. If you want your children to eat better, try to eat better yourself (at least when they are around). Let them see you eat with relish and restraint (even if you have to fake it). Pick blackberries together until your fingers are inky-purple. Present spinach as a delicious pancake-filling rather than a chore.

For parents struggling with their own chaotic patterns of eating – not to mention the day-to-day struggle of putting food on the table – all this can be immensely difficult. If you are lucky, the act of feeding children as well as yourself may be a fresh start. Seek help with your own eating, if you need it, and aim to be as kind to yourself with food as you are to them.

4

Guilt doesn't make us eat better, nor does it help us to feed better. Don't recriminate yourself about the way you fed them when they were babies. It's what happens next that matters and there's always another chance. Tomorrow is another breakfast.

5

The fact that a child doesn't like something now is not necessarily a sign that they will never like it. It may not feel like it, when you are trapped in an epic battle of wills over an omelette, but most children are very malleable when it comes to taste.

Over the past ten years, researchers and clinicians have pioneered a new technique for introducing children to new tastes. Dr Lucy Cooke of University College London, who has used it to teach hundreds of children to enjoy once-feared vegetables, calls it 'Tiny Tastes'. It sounds too simple to be true. The basic idea is that if you persuade children to try new foods in a minuscule dose – as small as a pea, or even a grain of rice – it's possible to try it multiple times without making the experience so unpleasant that they turn against the new food even more. Dr Cooke (author of *Stress-Free Feeding*) has found that if a child tries something ten to fourteen times on consecutive days, hate usually turns to love. If not, at least you gave it your best shot. The reward of a sticker helps, if your child is young enough. This method (minus the stickers) works with adults too, if you are open to trying.

6

It helps to recognize that some children are much harder to feed than others. I had no idea how fraught the basic matter of getting food from bowl to mouth could be until my third child was born with a cleft palate and he and I both came unstuck at mealtimes. Whether because of my stress or his reluctance, it was completely different from feeding my older two. He is 7 and new dishes still sometimes provoke tears (usually his). But we had it easy compared to families where the children are extremely selective eaters (in some cases, so selective that they have to be fed by a tube just to get enough calories to survive). There are toddlers who are scared of lumps and others of any food that isn't yellow. This is not the parents' fault – but with the right clinical support, a parent can help a child to rebuild their relationship with food. If you think your child is a selective eater, my heart goes out to you. Don't listen to the onlookers who make 'helpful' comments about how 'fussiness' is a modern form of self-indulgence and seek help from a qualified dietician.

7

When it comes to a child's likes and dislikes, nothing beats the power of exposure. Most of what we think of as personal taste is really memory. When babies were born to mothers who drank a lot of carrot juice while pregnant, they actively preferred the flavour of carrot-tasting cereal when taking their first bites of solid food, because they recognized it. Carrots tasted like home.

8

As parents, we underestimate our own power to influence a child's palate. *Anything* – no matter how sour or bitter – can start to taste good if you have enough positive memories of being fed it by a beloved parent.

9

If you want children to have varied palates, start them early on a variety of flavours. Baby books often tell you to wean babies onto sweet bland flavours like pumpkin, baby rice and sweet potato, because children love sweetness. I did this myself. A better plan might be to offer them a wider spectrum of bitter and sour vegetables – cauliflower, courgette, broccoli – right from the first bites. When bitter vegetables are offered to a 6-month-old the baby will often make the most dramatic expressions of horror and woe. 'Ignore the face,' says psychologist and feeding expert Dr Lucy Cooke. The grimace is just a physiological response. Adults still pucker their mouths at the taste of lemon, but it doesn't mean we hate citrus. When a baby really wants to tell you that they hate something, they will turn away, shake their head or clamp their mouth shut. This really does mean 'No' and should be respected.

10

Use the 'flavour window' to your advantage. Between the ages of 4 and 7 months, babies seem to be extraordinarily receptive to new flavours. This is a great moment to familiarize a baby with more bitter or challenging vegetables, as many kinds as possible.

11

The art of feeding is not pushing 'one more bite' into someone's mouth, however healthy the food. It is about creating a mealtime environment where those eating are free to develop their own tastes, because all the choices on the table are fine. Advocates of the 'Baby Led Weaning' system (BLW) say that children can be in charge of their own food choices from the very beginning. Gill Rapley is a British midwife who felt dissatisfied with the conventional wisdom that babies should be introduced to food via purées, given from a spoon. Rapley pioneered BLW, a method designed to be introduced at 6 months. You simply place chunks of normal (unsalted) food in front of the baby: steamed vegetables, soft pear; later, pieces of toast or even lamb chops. The baby will either grab it and attempt to eat – or not. BLW isn't the one true way to feed a child, because nothing ever is. But what we could all borrow from BLW is the idea that a child needs freedom to do their own learning about food.

12

Weaning them off milk is one thing. But the real task for a parent is to wean children off needing you.

13

No parent ever wins a food fight. Mealtimes become far more enjoyable all round when they are conducted on win–win lines rather than as a battle. Ideally, you will build up a repertoire of dishes your children positively enjoy that you can also feel positive about them eating. In our family, almond waffles – whether for breakfast or dessert – have healed many wounds. To me, they are a high-protein snack and not too sugary as things go. To the children, they are a vanilla-scented treat. Everyone – for once – is reconciled.

Win–win waffles

A child who eats a few of these will have consumed half an egg and the equivalent of a handful of almonds. These waffles are high in calcium, protein and fat. Given the new thinking on saturated fats, I see this as a good thing, because fat is both nourishing and filling. I notice that on the mornings I make these, my 7-year-old is not quite so rabidly hungry at the school gates when I pick him up. If you don't have a waffle maker, you can use the same mixture to make small American-style pancakes (cook for 1–2 minutes a side in a hot pan) but they won't be quite as good.

Serves 4 hungry people
80g unsalted butter, melted
20g caster sugar
2 large eggs
100g plain flour (I've made it with gluten-free flour for
    coeliac friends and it works fine)
80g ground almonds
1 teaspoon baking powder
170ml whole milk (or almond or coconut milk if you'd
    rather)
1 teaspoon good vanilla extract

Preheat the waffle maker. Put all the ingredients in a jug and blitz with a hand-held blender. Make the waffles as per the instructions for your machine. Be careful not to overfill or you get a batter volcano. I find 2 minutes about right, or until they are buff-coloured and crisp (but with a tiny bit of squidge in the centre). Serve with maple syrup (I measure out a little dipping pot for each child to stop them drenching half a bottle on a single waffle) and fresh fruit: chopped bananas, blackberries or sliced nectarines are all good.

14

If you want to know what foods to avoid giving to your child, start with almost everything marketed as 'kids' food'. It will likely be something that offers a very strange and unhealthy education in what food is and will train a child to expect everything to taste sweet, or salty, or both. It doesn't matter if it says 'one of your five-a-day' on the label or 'paediatrician-approved', it is probably still junk. Example: the sugariest of all the breakfast cereals are those in the kids' aisle. It's a disgrace that food manufacturers palm off such poor quality food on children, who depend on good nutrition to grow and develop.

FIVE UNHELPFUL FOODS MARKETED AT CHILDREN

Baby purées in pouches. For some reason, these have taken on aspirational middle-class overtones, maybe because the contents are often 'organic'. They tend to be made up of strange, sickly combinations such as sweet potato and blueberry, which would almost never be encountered in a real meal. And squeezing food direct from pouch to mouth is a terrible idea. It gives the child no opportunity to learn how to chew, which is actually a pretty useful skill to crack, eating-wise.

Fruit rolls. Yes, I know they often come with a cute collectable card and claim to be nothing but pure fruit. But they are basically candy and definitely no substitute for a fresh apple or pear. If you want to give your child sweets it's better if both you and the child understand that's what you are doing. In our house – I borrowed this idea from a wise friend – Friday is sweet day. I give them each a very small ramekin and they can fill it with whatever sweets they like, from the jar. Dentists say it's better for teeth if you eat sweets all in one go and then stop, rather than coating your mouth in them continuously.

Any product that comes with a free toy inside or a cartoon character on the label. This teaches a child that food is essentially boring and needs the distraction of entertainment to go down.

Anything marketed as 'suitable for lunchboxes'. These are usually laced with processed cheese and/or sugar and are strange quasi-foods.

All breakfast cereals sold as being specially for children. Part of me feels sad to say it, because as a child I loved the brightly coloured company of the cereal packet on the breakfast table. I've reached a compromise of allowing my kids a separate 'Saturday cereal'. The rest of the time they have porridge or some relatively unsweetened cereal like Shredded Wheat.

15

Serve vegetables first, when the appetite is keenest. Psychologists have found that serving 5-year-olds vegetables such as raw peppers before their main meal greatly increases the amount they eat. My once-picky 7-year-old became far more enthusiastic about vegetables when I started giving him a separate saucerful of them, before the main course. Now, we almost never have to prompt him to have the veg, which amazes me when I think back to the maelstrom of emotions that used to be unleashed by a single celery stick.

16

Girls eat better when food stops being something forbidden.

For some reason, parents seem to be more likely to keep a tight rein on what girls eat than with boys. It might be because mothers do most of the feeding and you are more likely to project your own fears about food and weight onto a child of the same sex.

Whatever the reason, restricting a girl's diet too stringently does not end well. Apart from making girls feel unhappy and body-conscious, pressuring a girl about her eating tends to backfire. One study involving nearly 200 5–7-year-old American girls and their mothers found that the girls whose mothers were most controlling about food were also more likely to overeat when given free access to snack foods such as pretzels, potato chips, popcorn and chocolate chip cookies. We want what we are told we can't have.

17

Instead of encouraging your girl (or boy) to obsess about 'bad foods' or changing her weight, it would be more productive to teach her how to recognize her own hunger and fullness. Up until the age of 3–4, a child has a natural instinct about how much to eat and will eat just the right amount, even if served a large portion. After this age, the skill is lost. Luckily it can be retaught. Paediatrician Susan Johnson worked with a group of 4–5-year-olds in a nursery, asking them to play with dolls who had different 'stomachs' filled with salt. Some of the dolls had empty stomachs, some were half-full and some were completely full. At snack-time, the children were asked to put their hands over their own stomachs and to compare them with the dolls' stomachs as they ate. After six weeks of this game, the children would spontaneously say things like, 'I'm not hungry any more so I'm going to stop eating.' We could recreate this game at the family dinner table. Without moralizing about it, encourage your children to make the connection between what they eat and the feeling in their bellies.

18

Boys eat better when their parents continue to expect them to eat vegetables and include them in home-cooked meals as they get older. Better still, get them to prepare the home-cooked meals themselves.

The strange idea persists that boys need different foods from girls: meatier, manlier and in bigger portions. It's true that levels of exercise and size being roughly equal, boys need a little more energy than girls (but not if it's a girl who plays hockey five times a week and a boy who plays computer games five hours a day). But our culture stokes boys with dangerous delusions about just how much energy they need. In many countries, parents show a strange favouritism to boys by not expecting them to eat as many vegetables as girls. This is not really doing them a favour. In Thailand, girls eat many more fruits and vegetables than boys, which is reflected in obesity rates: twice as many Thai boys as girls are obese. In Britain, too, the trend is for boys to eat declining quantities of fruits and vegetables (and far from declining quantities of burgers and chips). Even if we think we are beyond such sexist notions, it's easy to make subliminal assumptions about boys 'needing' great wodges of meat and carbs and not requiring anything so girlish as green leaves. The biggest nutritional favour you can do for your boys is to teach them a love of salad. The secret to enjoying salad, as anyone knows, is the right dressing.

Salad for a boy

This dressing makes any green leaf taste almost addictive. It's creamy and garlicky: a little bit like bottled ranch dressing but so much better. Even a 5-year-old boy can learn how to shake it up in a jam jar.

Serves 4

2 tablespoons whole-milk yoghurt

2 tablespoons olive oil

½ clove garlic, peeled, crushed or grated on a
    Microplane grater

a big pinch of Maldon sea salt

a small pinch of sugar

¼ teaspoon Dijon mustard

1 teaspoon apple or white wine vinegar

1 teaspoon lemon juice

(or use all lemon juice if you prefer)

Add all the ingredients to a clean jam jar. Screw on the lid and shake. Use a piece of lettuce to taste it. You might want more salt or lemon, or even a dash of water, if you find it too thick. If you love the pungency of raw garlic, add more. Use it to dress any combination of leaves and other raw vegetables, toss and serve. Examples: torn romaine, cress and spinach; watercress, Little Gem and red radicchio; sliced raw mushrooms, sliced radishes, rocket and soft round lettuce. Wash and dry the leaves well.

I haven't yet met a child who didn't get a kick out of using a salad spinner. Delegate the washing of lettuce as soon as you can.

For total salad refuseniks, you could use the dressing as a dipping sauce for raw carrot sticks.

19

Girls should eat man food. The single greatest nutritional deficit in our diets right now is the iron deficiency of girls. Yet we hardly talk about it. Across the globe, rich or poor, fat or thin, millions of adolescent girls are anaemic because they do not have enough iron-rich foods in their diet to cover the leap in what their bodies need – from 8mg to 15mg – when they start to menstruate. Many more have iron depletion, where no iron is stored in the body, which can cause tiredness, headaches and impaired cognitive function.

Around half of British girls are also low in zinc and magnesium. Too many overweight teenage girls are being pressurized by their families to lose weight when what they in fact need is better nourishment (which would almost certainly help them to lose weight along the way). Iron-deprived girls of every size need to be 'built up', as the reassuring old phrase had it, with soft-boiled eggs and wholemeal toast soldiers; with dark leafy greens; steak; and hearty Tuscan bean soup. In short, these girls need man food.

SIX IRON-RICH FOODS
WORTH LEARNING TO LOVE

Pistachio nuts
All nuts are rich in iron, but pistachios have the most.

Lentils
A serving of Puy lentils contains about 4g iron.

Mussels
A bowl of *moules marinières* contains as much as 7g iron and they are surprisingly cheap and easy to cook.

Black treacle – around 7mg in 2 tablespoons
Make sticky dark gingerbread for an after-school snack.

Dark green leaves, from chard to kale to spinach
All contain iron to varying degrees. Your body will find it easier to absorb the iron if you combine plant sources of iron with some vitamin C. A squeeze of lemon should do it.

Sesame seeds
Tahini sauce – sesame paste diluted with lemon juice, water and salt – is a delicious iron-rich addition to almost any plate of steamed vegetables.

Spiced chicken livers for a girl

I first got this idea from Tamasin Day-Lewis, but have
adapted the spices. Lots of people think they can't
and won't like liver. But once you develop a taste for
it, the rich moussy texture and slightly mineral
flavour is comforting. Since the liver is the part of the
body that processes toxins, it's definitely worth
seeking out organic chicken livers. (Waitrose has
them.) They are still astonishingly good value
compared to almost any other meat.

Serves 3

3 teaspoons panch phoran (this 5-spice blend of
  whole seeds is easy to get at Asian grocers; or if
  you can't find it, use 1 teaspoon each whole cumin
  seeds, nigella seeds and black mustard seeds)
¾ teaspoon Maldon sea salt
½ teaspoon black peppercorns
1 tablespoon plain flour
2 tablespoons olive oil
1 large onion, halved and sliced
400g organic chicken livers
10g butter
To serve: flatbreads or pitta, whole-milk plain
  yoghurt, lemon, watercress

Heat the panch phoran in a small frying pan over a gentle heat until fragrant and starting to pop – about a minute. Tip the seeds into a pestle and mortar, add the salt and peppercorns and crush, not too fine. Mix with the flour and set aside. Meanwhile, heat 1 tablespoon of the oil and fry the onion, stirring now and then, until golden. Trim the livers by cutting each lobe in half and then in half again, removing any connecting strands. Dredge them in the flour-spice mix. Heat the rest of the oil and all the butter in a large frying pan. Put the livers in and cook without turning for 2 minutes or so until crisp on one side. Turn and cook for another minute or so on the other side. Test one. You want them pink but not oozingly red. Serve, with the fried onions, warm flatbread or pitta, whole-milk plain yoghurt, wedges of lemon and watercress (which boosts the iron content of the meal even more, as well as cutting the richness of the liver with its sprightly green).

Black bean chilli for a girl

Every teenager I've tried this on was mad about this dark, spicy chilli. Black beans and lentils are both a superb source of iron so I feel happy when my 13-year-old daughter eats a bowlful of this for supper. I don't make it super-hot because you can always add more chilli at the table. I prefer chilli without tinned tomatoes, which can add a muddy taste. This hearty chilli is equally good with flatbreads or rice.

Serves 4, with leftovers

3 tablespoons olive oil

1 large red onion, peeled and chopped

3 cloves garlic, peeled and chopped

1 thumb of ginger, grated

1 heaped teaspoon ground cumin

1 heaped teaspoon ground cinnamon

2 teaspoons chipotle paste

4 sweet potatoes, peeled and cubed

100g Puy lentils

1 teaspoon Maldon sea salt

2 x 400g tins black beans (or 250g dried black beans, soaked and cooked)

4 large vine tomatoes, chopped

500ml water

juice of ½ lime

To serve: limes, sour cream, chilli sauce, sliced
     avocados, flatbreads/rice/baked potatoes

Heat the oil in a big pan or casserole and cook the
onion until translucent, about 5 minutes. Add the
garlic and ginger and sauté for a couple more minutes
or until fragrant. Add the spices and chipotle paste
and stir for a few seconds before adding the sweet
potatoes, lentils and salt. Stir for a minute before
adding the beans (including their liquid), tomatoes
and water. Simmer with the lid on for 20 minutes.
Then remove the lid and cook for another 10–20
minutes or until the sweet potatoes are tender and
most of the liquid has evaporated. If it becomes too
dry at any point, add more water. Taste for seasoning
and add the juice of half a lime. Serve in bowls, letting
people help themselves to lime, sour cream, chilli
sauce, avocado, along with flatbreads or rice or baked
potatoes.

20

Feeding children can start to feel so stressful and complicated that the joy of sharing food gets lost. If you manage to teach your child that meals are fun and that real food – in all its variety – is to be enjoyed, you are doing all right. When all else fails, try sitting on the floor and having a picnic. A friend of mine used to lay a tablecloth on the floor and sit with her daughter, sharing a plate of globe artichokes, a loaf of bread and a bowl of mayonnaise. They dipped the artichokes in the mayonnaise, tore off hunks of bread and sat together as companions sharing a feast.

MAKING CHANGES

Vanya: To begin a new life – tell me, how should I begin? Where do I start?
Astrov: Oh get away with you. New life indeed.
Chekhov, Uncle Vanya

1

If you want yourself to eat better, focus less on the food and more on your own response to it.

2

We all have mixed feelings about change. If you were not ambivalent about changing your diet, you wouldn't have picked up this book. A person can passionately want to lose weight but equally passionately desire the comfort of five slices of soft white bread with chocolate spread. I can't pretend that there are no downsides to learning to eat less. There are just so many times in a day that you have to say 'No'. But the part of you that wants *not* to eat five pieces of bread is also real. Try to listen to your own desire for change and repeat it to yourself before you can talk yourself out of it. Over a long career, dietician Dympna Pearson has seen many people whose health will be seriously jeopardized without a change in diet, including diabetics who risk losing a leg if they don't reduce their sugar consumption and coeliacs who can't stick to a gluten-free diet. Pearson finds that when clients first see her they might say, 'I want to, but I can't.' She knows they will only actually change when she hears them say not, 'I wish I could', but 'I will'.

3

A small change to how you eat isn't small if it sticks.

One bowl of soup or plate of salad on a Monday lunchtime may not mean much, but a whole year of good Monday lunches is a paradigm shift.

Sometimes – especially if you have a lot of weight to lose – every tiny effort feels futile. How much difference can one meal make? Hang in there. Research suggests that it takes an average of sixty-six days, or a bit over two months, for a new habit to stick. This can feel like for ever if you are still on day 23. But if you can make it through to day 66, you might just get over the hill, to the easy plains where the new habit is second nature.

4

When making tweaks to your diet, try to avoid the mindset of deprivation. Except for the odd coffee shop treat, I recently switched from milky lattes to black coffee. Instead of feeling sad that I wasn't drinking all that lovely foamy milk, I would ask myself whether I'd rather have a drink of water or a drink of black coffee. I chose the black coffee. It then tasted so much nicer. Giving up sugar in tea is one of the habits that many struggle to break. But if you can stick with it for long enough – without substituting sweeteners, which only trick your palate – the old sugary tea genuinely starts to taste sickly rather than comforting. These small 'micro-habits' are good ones to experiment with. If you can prove to yourself that you can enjoy something as habitual as tea in a less sweet form, what's to stop you from changing more of your tastes?

5

The great thing about *not* being on a diet is that you can't break it. Setbacks are to be expected when you are trying to change for good. If you suddenly find yourself slipping into old habits of compulsive or emotional eating, try to analyse what provoked you so that you can prepare yourself next time. Were you upset? Tired? Angry? Sleep-deprived? At a family gathering? All of the above? You almost certainly won't be able to avoid all these triggers, but it helps if you can at least recognize what drove you to put the food in your mouth. When you start regretting something you've eaten, I also find it helps if you tell yourself it was actually allowed. No amount of 'shoulds' will change the fact that you did eat it, whatever it was. It's gone. Permission granted. If you consumed something your diet supposedly didn't allow, don't blame yourself, blame the diet.

6

If you want to learn new tastes, salt could be your friend, at least at first. It's the familiar savour that binds a plate of food together. We have been taught to fear salt, and see it as a poison that will give you a stroke or heart disease. But new scientific evidence published in *The Lancet* in 2016 by epidemiologist Andrew Mente suggests that eating too little sodium (under 1.5g a day) can be at least as bad for your health as eating too much. The majority of salt in the average diet comes from processed food. If you have seriously cut down on processed foods (including breakfast cereals, some of which contain a gram of sodium in a single bowl), you can afford to add a little salt back in, assuming you don't have high blood pressure. Mente surveyed data from more than 130,000 people across 49 countries and found that consuming more than 6mg of sodium a day, a very high amount (think two extra-large tubs of salty cinema popcorn), was indeed linked to greater risk of mortality. But Mente also found that a moderate intake of 3–5mg a day seemed to carry no health risks for people with normal blood pressure. It's definitely possible to reduce your palate for salt, simply by cutting back in increments, but to me, salt in moderation is miraculous stuff. It enhances sweetness and takes the edge off bitterness and makes everything moreish, even beetroot. Think of a slice of rye bread spread with unsalted butter and covered in juicy slices of tomato. This is a pleasant enough snack. Add salt, though, and it becomes something to crave (and the potassium in the tomato balances the sodium in the salt).

7

Blur the boundaries of 'healthy' and 'unhealthy' food. We all put food in certain categories. Chefs know that you can get customers to order certain unfamiliar ingredients by pairing them with something homely and beloved such as mashed potatoes. We could use the same trick on ourselves. If you think of bacon and eggs as pleasure and broccoli as rabbit-food, you could try broccoli *with* bacon instead.

8

Children learn to eat better when the process feels less like a lecture and more like a game. The same is true for adults.

9

Disgust is even more powerful than desire. We should use this more to our advantage. The ideal scenario for healthy food shopping is when you won't buy most of what's for sale, not because you shouldn't, but because it repels you. Psychologist Paul Rozin has found that – perhaps unsurprisingly – almost no one wants to eat a box of chocolates if someone else has taken a bite out of each one first. If you see each hamburger shop as a temptation, life will be hard, because there are just so many darned hamburger shops. If you can train yourself to notice some of the ways in which fast food is disgusting – the grease, the sickly sweetness – it's easier to say 'No' without even thinking about it.

10

Be prepared to adjust your diet and tastes for different phases of life. As you age, you may need to eat less of some foods and more of others. To take just one example, there are signs that over the age of 50 we may need more protein than before, to counteract the loss of muscle mass as we age. It's easy to cling on to old food habits long after they have ceased to be useful. Just because your diet appeared to work fine at 20 does not mean that the same foods will feed you equally well decades later.

11

Regular exercise definitely helps: the endorphins, the expenditure of energy, the fact you are doing something other than eating. But again, find a version that you like so much you positively want to do it, rather than the one that burns the most fat but leaves you so drained you need to take urgent solace in carbohydrates. It took me far longer to warm up to exercise than to healthy eating. I imagine I felt about running as some people do about cabbage. I heard fitness enthusiasts talking about a 'runner's high' or doing triathlons at the weekend and felt baffled and slightly threatened. Then – very late in the day – I joined a gym and discovered that yoga classes could (for me) actually be fun if they didn't go on too long and the teacher wasn't too bossy. I also started doing work-outs, but in tiny tastes, as if trying a strange new ingredient. Sometimes, I stopped after just ten minutes. No matter – it was ten minutes more than I'd ever done since PE lessons at school. Gradually, I found myself wanting to do it for longer. Listening to music helped. Now, I am doing a brilliant free NHS app called Couch to 5K that is designed to get you running 5K in nine weeks. An encouraging woman talks to you as you run and tells you not to give up. You don't need to run in a gym – a park is fine.

Confession: I've been stuck on week 6 for over a year. But that's OK.

12

Make exercise – in whatever form you can fit into your life – its own reward. Don't exercise to punish yourself for the treats you ate or to get abs of steel. Think of it as time away from all the hassles and demands of modern life. No one can expect you to answer an email or find the kitchen scissors when you are in plank pose.

13

Ignore those who say it isn't worth exercising because you can't 'outrun a bad diet'. In most recent studies, exercise alone (as against changing diet) comes out very poorly as an intervention for losing weight. But in real life as opposed to studies, you don't have to choose exercise or diet. You can choose both.

Whether or not it helps you lose weight, exercise has some pretty remarkable side effects, ranging from improving the symptoms of anxiety and depression to improving heart health and giving you healthier microbes in your gut. Some of the most interesting evidence on the benefits of exercise concerns people who have succeeded in losing large amounts of weight without regaining it. Numerous studies confirm that these people tend to engage in regular exercise. Exercise may or may not help you to lose weight, but it certainly helps you not to regain it, which is the harder part.

14

Changing our diets always involves losses as well as gains. It helps to be honest with yourself about this. The water is cold when you first dip a toe in the pool. Giving up junk food involves a separation from some of your fondest childhood memories. Learning to like new foods can feel like leaving your old self behind. The best you can do is to get past your own mixed feelings and try again. The hardest thing, after so many false starts and wrong turns, is finding the motivation to get back in the pool and stay there long enough to get acclimatized.

15

Don't take diet advice from your scales. It's easy to fall into the trap of thinking that you should celebrate losing 5 pounds with a slap-up meal; or conversely, that you are not 'allowed' a slice of birthday cake because you haven't reached your target weight. On adverts, we only ever see skinny people eating. But large or small, everyone needs and deserves food.

16

The wonderful secret of being an omnivore is that we can adjust our desires, even late in the game. In this godforsaken world of wars and taxes, there are many things we cannot change. Luckily, the majority of our own food habits do not fall into this category. Our tastes are learned in the context of immense social influences, whether from our family, our friends, or the cheery font on a bottle of soda. Yet no matter what our age, it's always possible to carve out new tastes for ourselves.

17

Pleasure will get you there quicker than denial.

18

Expect your emotions to change along with your diet. Overeating is an effective way to silence anger and fear. Without the analgesic of excess carbs, you may experience furies you didn't know you had in you. This is not necessarily bad: to know your real feelings is better than to suppress them. But it can be a shock.

19

Some say changing your diet in radical ways isn't possible. To those people I say: look at Japan. The Japanese now have an enviably balanced relationship with food: very low rates of obesity coupled with a deeply pleasurable attitude to eating. It's easy to assume that there's something innate and deeply Japanese that helps them to eat this way. But the wonderful cuisine that we think of as 'Japanese food' has only existed for a few decades. After the Second World War, the Japanese quite rapidly changed their diet, becoming more open to new flavours and cooking techniques. For centuries, the Japanese ate a much worse diet than their neighbours in Korea and China. Even in the early twentieth century, they did not have the spicy katsu curries and ramen noodles that we now think of as so typically Japanese. People sat in silence at the dinner table, rather than noisily enjoying plates of soba noodles and sushi as they do now.

We should be encouraged by the example of Japan. Under the right conditions, a whole country can change the way it eats. And you can change too.

20

Find new activities that have nothing to do with food. Part of our trouble with eating is that we expect too much of it, turning to the fridge as a form of diversion (the Tony Soprano syndrome). Fill your evenings with more interesting outlets for your appetites and food need not loom quite so large. Sad books and funny films work for me.

21

You know you have really changed not when you have reached a certain size but when your eating doesn't feel broken any more. The word health originally meant 'whole' or complete. To be healthy (the old word was 'hale') was to be sound of mind and body. Many of us – whether we diet or not – have lost that wholeness with our eating. But it's never too late to pick up the pieces and attempt to put them back together.

ACKNOWLEDGEMENTS

This is a short book, but it benefited from the knowledge and experience of many others. Food, I find, is a near-universal topic of conversation and many of the things I have learned have come from chance encounters, some virtual, some real, with people who won't realize how much they helped. Although this is not a scholarly book, it does draw on the research and wisdom of many experts in the field of nutrition and the psychology of eating and in particular I'd like to mention the work of Lucy Cooke, Paul Rozin, Keith Williams, Tim Lang, Corinna Hawkes, Theresa Marteau, Tim Spector, Julie Mennella and Gary Beauchamp.

I've learned at least as much from reading cookery writers; there are too many to list them all here, but they include Diana Henry, Mark Bittman, Anna Jones, Marlena Spieler, Jacob Kenedy, Claudia Roden, Lucas Hollweg, Olia Hercules and Meera Sodha. My thinking on food is always sharpened by my friends and colleagues at the Oxford Symposium on Food & Cookery. For various conversations about eating and its pathologies, I owe special thanks to Emily Wilson, Catherine Blyth, Martha Repp, Miranda Landgraf, Ranjita Lohan and Lisa Runciman. I'm grateful to Tom Runciman for reading the manuscript, to Tasha Runciman for being the best kitchen companion and to Leo Runciman for demanding almond waffles at regular intervals. I'm thankful, as always, for the judgment and support of my agents, Sarah Ballard and Zoe Pagnamenta. I am fortunate to have worked with Louise Haines, an inspiring editor and a wise voice on food, and would also like to thank the rest of the team at 4th Estate including the brilliant Patrick Hargadon, Sarah Thickett and Jo Walker.

FIRST BITE:
How we learn to eat

Bee Wilson

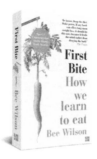

An exploration of the extraordinary and surprising origins of our taste and eating habits, in *First Bite* award-winning food writer Bee Wilson explains how we can change our palates to lead healthier, happier lives.

'A brilliant, heartfelt book about this crisis in our contemporary diet . . . Wilson is intelligent, passionate, sincere, tirelessly curious and endlessly willing to admit mistakes and learn from experience'
John Lanchester

4th ESTATE · *London*